MW00951889

IMPORTANT INFORMATION

WHAT THIS BOOK IS NOT!

Whilst I have referred where appropriate to important medically based studies, books and medical papers, this book has not been written as a medical research paper, designed to cover dozens of scientific subjects.

I have deliberately avoided the current trend in many diet books to constantly cherry pick medical and scientific studies to support the book's conclusions. This book is not intended as a reference item to satisfy those readers that might be looking for useful research material.

This book is about a real life journey and the real life testing processes that have identified the most effective ways to develop great eating behaviours and incorporating those behaviours into our daily food choices.

There will be a detailed bibliography attached to this book. This is a truly exciting and rapidly evolving science and there is a vast amount of material to read and study about Epigenetics and Functional Medicine in general, especially in the way that these insights apply to intelligent weight management. If you require further information, I suggest you contact me for specific recommendations at beranparry@gmail.com

FREE PERSONALISED EATING BEHAVIOUR TEST

http://www.skinnydeliciouslife.com/take-the-skinny-delicious-smart-genetic-eating-behaviour-test/

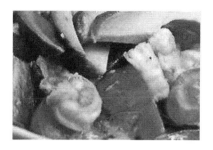

THE PALEO EPIGENETIC

COOKBOOK

By

BERAN PARRY

Edited by

GREG PARRY PHD

Contents

Acknowledgements for the Epigenetic Eating Programs.

The inspiration to write this book began more than thirty years ago when I embarked on my first nutritional science courses under the tutelage of Dr Boris Chaitow in South Africa. During the past three decades, I have been most fortunate to receive the guidance, teachings and encouragement of some immensely talented and dedicated doctors and professors. It has been a fascinating journey of exploration, the pathway lit by the giants of natural medicine and naturopathic nutrition. More recently, my studies in the field of Functional Medicine have proved immensely helpful and I would like to pay tribute to the genius, courage and dedication of the following specialists who have assisted me enormously in my quest to share the life-changing knowledge contained in this book.

Among them are Dr Boris Chaitow, Debra Waterhouse, Dr Christiane Northrup, Dr Carolyne Dean, Dr Vasant Lad, Dr Mona Lisa Shulz, Dr Loren Cordain, Dr Patrick Vercammen and Dr Ron Grisanti.

I would particularly like to acknowledge the shining inspiration of a truly remarkable doctor who has been a constant source of knowledge, encouragement and inspiration. Dr Ann Lannoye, a Functional Medicine Specialist and member of the Institute of Functional Medicine, has been a most generous and tireless source of knowledge and enthusiasm for the benefits of Functional Medicine. She provided the inspiration to link my nutritional and eating behaviour work with the Functional Diagnostic Medicine and the analysis of Epigenetic Expression. Dr Lannoye's extensive knowledge and scientific rigour have been one of the major cornerstones of our next book about Functional Medicine in which I hope to have Dr Lannoye join me as a contributor and authority.

My functional medicine research and its conclusions have been so fundamental to my understanding of intelligent nutrition, that I undertook studies at the Functional Medicine University in South Carolina. Dr Ron Grisanti has been a most generous provider of case study information in these vitally important subjects.

I am also delighted to announce a series of further projects with Dr Ann Lannoye and Greg Parry PhD, also based in the field of Functional Medicine. We are scheduling a series of international seminars, professional training courses and wellbeing conventions. If you would like to know more go to...

www.beranparry.com

Preface

Let's talk about food! Do you love to eat? Do you really enjoy your food? Join the club! Most of us take great pleasure from our daily sustenance but did you know that certain foods can really help to heal your body more effectively than conventional medicines? We're learning to recognise more and more that good food really is nature's finest medicine. But you need to make sure you're choosing exactly the right kind of food for your body. And now the complete formula for boosting your health and wellbeing is finally available- right at your fingertips. Welcome to the ultimate Paleo Recipe Book, 420 fabulous meal recommendations, 365 mouth-watering recipes, 12 weeks of life-enhancing Paleo Daily Meal Planners, 12 Categories of Recipe Plans. This is your dedicated Paleo Epigenetic Resource, specifically designed to help you to restore your body to its best possible condition.

As a nutritionist specialising in the revolutionary field of functional medicine and Paleo Diet Systems, I advise people every day about the best foods they can eat to prevent, treat and even reverse chronic disease. We focus on foods that are packed with nutrients, the essential energy sources that our bodies crave to promote total health and well-being. But food choice and diets are complicated areas that can produce a great deal of unnecessary confusion. One of the challenges when working within this complex area is the contradictory information that's often published by well-meaning enthusiasts. You can read for instance that a Vegan diet is great for weight loss, that it can reverse diabetes and lower cholesterol. But studies report similar results for the Paleo diet books that fill our bookshelves. The problem is that researchers are often highly selective about the data they report. They look for the evidence that will support their conclusions or philosophies. No wonder things can get a little confusing!

But help is at hand. The 365 Paleo Epigenetic Diet Revolution features the best elements from both the Vegan and Paleo systems and delivers great results not just in terms of weight control but also as a powerful enhancement to total wellbeing.

Introduction

We live in an incredibly busy world with so many distractions screaming for our attention that it's a miracle that we get anything done at all. And then we're supposed to create space in an already over-crowded day to provide for the needs of our bodies. We're expected to know somehow what's healthy and then avoid the temptations of easy, quick, convenience foods. No wonder the world is experiencing an explosion in obesity rates. We make life much so more difficult than it needs to be. But that challenge is finally over.

Help is at hand. Real help. Practical, easy, no-nonsense help that will help you take care of the essential issue of eating healthily every single day of your life. And that is how this book came into being.

My three decades of experience as a certified nutritionist with a background in functional medicine enabled me to identify the daily problem that so many patients experienced. They really struggled to find the time to plan meals and source the right ingredients. So I decided to take the strain out of the process and build this fabulous collection of intelligent eating recipes into easy-to-follow meal plans that would just make your life so much easier. A handy reference guide to take care of all the decision making steps of organising the best possible nutrition. Boosting your health. Turning up your happiness. Every single day.

I want you to feel better than ever. I want you to discover the joys of living with your ideal weight. I want your energy and health levels to soar. And I want the process to be as easy, comfortable and delicious as possible. I want you to enjoy the journey.

The 365 Paleo Epigenetic Diet Revolution Recipe Book is your new friend and helper, your constant companion and guide on the pathway to total wellness. I offer it with love and my belief in your right and ability to live a truly wonderful life. It begins right here.

Chapter 1

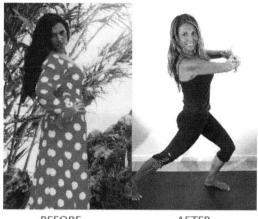

BEFORE   AFTER

My Story

Welcome to the start of a whole new way of life! We're about to embark on an adventure together and my job is to help and guide you on your new pathway to the health, weight and wellbeing of your dreams. My name is Beran Parry and for the past thirty-five years I've been studying, practising and advising thousands of people about truly effective nutrition and weight loss. A lot of this passion comes from my family background. Growing up in a family with major health and weight problems, I realised at a very early age that body shape, weight and health are all deeply connected. To complicate matters, I became pregnant at the tender age of 18 and I experienced all the dismay and daily disappointment of significant weight gain plus the frustration of struggling to get rid of the extra pounds after giving birth to my lovely son Christopher.

By the time I was twenty-two, more than thirty years ago, I began studying nutrition, exercise physiology, integrative medicine and holistic health. I was immensely fortunate to find myself studying at one of the early pioneering centres of Integrative Alternative Medicine. This was the world renowned High Rustenberg Hydro, set in the beautiful countryside around Stellenbosch University, not far from my birthplace, Cape Town, in South Africa.

I studied very intensively for four years under the guidance of various medical and homeopathic doctors whilst also studying banking and finance. My studies continued right up until 1986 when I moved from South Africa to Europe.

The happy story takes a tougher turn when I went through the trauma of divorce and promptly acquired an extra 20 kilos of weight! I really piled on the pounds in record time and battled so hard to lose every single ounce. I really do understand the challenges of effective and enduring, healthy weight loss!

Beran Moves to Europe!

As you might imagine, leaving my beautiful home in warm, sunny Cape Town and relocating to the cold and damp of northern Europe was not an easy process. The stress levels went off the chart and, well, I bet you can guess what happened. That's right. Those 20 kilos I'd worked so hard to lose came back with a vengeance. It was a fat-fuelled action replay of those dark days after my divorce. But it really made me wonder about the real connections between stress and unhealthy weight gain.

But life rarely follows a straight line and in 2000, my path took an unexpected detour when I was diagnosed with a serious health problem. It was my thyroid gland. This incredibly important little gland had produced a 6cm tumour that was growing and gradually blocking my windpipe. Not a happy discovery!

It was a turning point in my life and I realised in my heart that this time I really had to apply all my energies to the issues of health, weight control and wellbeing. This became my focal point. It grew into a passionate quest to share my knowledge and experience with as many people as possible. What started as a search for answers to my own health problems all those years ago became a quest to find universal principles that would apply to everyone. We made many changes from that point onwards and, as my health completely recovered, we discovered more insights into what really constitutes great health and profound wellbeing.

The range of interests broadened, encompassing naturopathic medicine, eating behaviours and disorders, orthomolecular medicine and the ancient Ayurvedic traditions that are witnessing a global revival after thousands of years of practise.

My studies and passions about wellbeing have now developed further into the incredible and exciting area of Functional Medicine and I am studying a Degree with the Functional Medicine University at present.

All these years of training, study, practise and experience are distilled and crystalised right here in your personal weight loss transformation workbook.

The reality is that I'm fitter and healthier today than at any other time in my life. Despite all the negative expectations surrounding the subjects of ageing and weight control, I can show you how to tame your body-fat problems and turn back the clock, helping you to find a younger, fitter, skinnier, stronger, healthier you. So let's get started!

Chapter 2

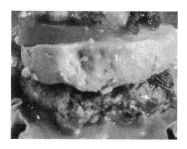

So Why Can't I Lose Weight? And why can't I keep the weight off?

These are good questions because even champion weight losers often put the weight back on, suffering the seemingly inevitable see-saw effect of cyclical weight loss followed by weight gain. Can we do something to correct this problem? Of course we can! That's exactly what this book is for.

1. Create Good Habits

Willpower - the mantra of the naturally thin. Why willpower alone is overrated

Let's just accept that we're going to need more than willpower to get the job done. When you rely on willpower alone you set yourself up for failure and disappointment. Routine and old habits are strongly embedded in our behaviour so they will win out over willpower 99% of the time and this is another reason why diets simply don't work. They rely on short-term changes that no normal person can ever hope to maintain.

A good habit doesn't require willpower or discipline. By definition, a habit is something you don't even think about. It's something that you do or feel automatically. Bad habits don't usually take up too much of your attention either until you begin to suffer the consequences. Because bad habits inevitably have a down side. If there's a habit you're trying to change, you need to be motivated to do something about it. Most of us respond positively to a suitable reward (not food!) to make the change worthwhile and repeatable.

2. Cravings

Intense hunger. Thin people can never understand this. It's a hard but inescapable fact. An overweight person is physically hungry more often than a naturally thin person. And the hunger is much more intense. Thin people frequently accuse overweight people of lacking the self-control to stop eating. It's a great story and it makes thin people feel better. But it is absolutely not true. Not. True. The thin person cannot possibly comprehend the intense physiological and almost constant hunger that overweight people have to deal with. It has nothing to do with self-control. This is a real, gnawing, overwhelming and intense physical hunger. That's a good reason why those very fortunate, naturally thin people and exercise gurus should not write books on how to lose weight. They have no concept of the scale and depth of the challenges that overweight people have to deal with on a daily basis. You have to know what those hunger drives really feel like before you start giving advice! One of the startling revelations that we're going to explore together is the fact that many overweight people are starving. Their bodies are starved of essential nutrients so they're constantly hungry and their bodies are crying out for something nutritiously worthwhile to satisfy those basic needs. It's so ironic that obese individuals feel so hungry but it's a reality that we're going to deal with by fixing the problem right at its source.

Eating when your body doesn't need the fuel.

Overweight people are also prone to problems with "emotional eating" or cravings. Certain food cravings fall into the above hunger category as they are certainly physiological in nature. Other food cravings or emotional eating occur when you are physically not hungry, but your hunger becomes a displacement activity to satisfy unfulfilled emotional needs. This hunger might be emotional in origin but it feels exactly like real physical hunger when you experience it.

3. Genetics.

There are thousands of diet books, countless weight-loss articles and hundreds of weight loss organisations but we all know about the real problem of losing weight; the fat begins to slip away, we post the good news on Facebook, celebrating the success - and then we see all the good work undone as we put the pounds back on in a very short period of time. Now that is just too frustrating!

Relax. Help is finally at hand. We'll show how to re-set your metabolism and take control of your weight issues for the rest of your life.

If you still suspect that your inherited DNA is responsible for making you overweight, I'd like to repeat that it's being proved time and time again that genetics simply do not play the only role in causing obesity. Genetics can be thanked for your general body shape but are not the main cause for a low metabolism, intense and constant physical hunger, or emotional eating. The answer lies in our behaviour and in our environment. In other words, our weight is entirely a product of what we do.

Do things differently and the weight ceases to be problem.

Excited? Stay with me. Read on!...We're just getting started!

SUMMARY

Metabolism is the key

Recognising intense hunger and cravings

Creating good habits

Managing your environment

Building support from friends, family and colleagues

Eliminating the villains from the weight loss narrative

Chapter 3

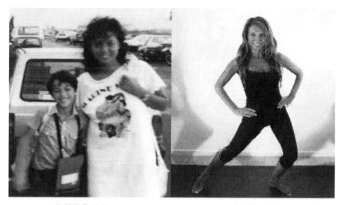

BEFORE   AFTER

The Paleo Diet and Epigenetics

The Paleo Diet

The theory is that many of our current health problems are a result of our modern eating habits. There's been a great deal of publicity surrounding the growing view that we simply haven't evolved to the point where we can safely consume a grain-rich diet. Our distant ancestors in the Old Stone Age or Paleolithic Era consumed a very different diet compared to modern humans because they simply didn't have access to agriculture. That's because agriculture didn't exist. It hadn't been invented. The typical caveman's food was natural, unprocessed, varied, seasonal and a result of labour-intensive, hunter-gathering activities.

The Paleo approach to nutrition recognises that we've only been consuming grains for the last ten thousand years or so. That's a long wait at the bus stop but it really is not long enough in evolutionary terms for humans to have adapted to this radical shift in eating behaviour. The modern diet is heavily reliant on grains and dairy products and suffers from a toxic surfeit of sugar. Grains were the mechanism that allowed for a more predictable food supply and those ancient crop surpluses provided the essential catalyst from which the seeds of civilisation sprang. The problem, as you now know only too well, is that grains damage the gut, weaken the immune system and degrade our health.

The Paleo alternative recognises how our digestive system works and focuses on providing the best quality fuel for our bodies. That includes fresh fruits, vegetables, lean meat, eggs and nuts. No grains. No processed sugars. No milk products. Paleo has scored very highly as a weight control mechanism because this kind of diet suits our evolutionary history so well. When we adapt our eating habits to this more natural way of getting our daily calories, our metabolisms shift from carb-burning to fat-burning. No surprise then that the Paleo diet has become a favourite tool for encouraging serious weight loss and for enhancing better levels of health.

The focus is on natural, unprocessed food and it is this emphasis on eating as naturally as possible that is the key to the method's success. As you might expect in a new way of approaching our food needs, the Paleo diet has spawned a number of variations and alternatives. Some enthusiasts avoid all forms of dairy produce whilst others are convinced that some specific dairy products are essential. The wisdom of avoiding grains though is widely accepted by most Paleo devotees.

The Epigenetic Eating Take on the Paleo Diet

You might recognise some aspects of the Paleo Diet in our advice in this book. It certainly has some interesting and relevant merits in terms of getting the body into great shape and the emphasis on pure protein and natural, unprocessed vegetables is a key to restoring the intestinal flora to its healthiest and most effective condition.

How the eating habits we acquired in the past profoundly affect our food choices today.

How Genetics are no longer the prime influence on our health and wellbeing

Epigenetics provides us with the insights, analysis, tools and strategies for permanent healthy weight loss.

Perhaps you've never heard about the excitement in medical and scientific circles about the latest revelations in the field of Epigenetics. But before we go any further, you're probably wondering what on earth Epigenetics really means. Is it contagious? Can we get it at the grocery store? Does it come in my size? So let's start by answering an important question: "What exactly is Epigenetics?"

The formal description of Epigenetics refers to the study of changes in organisms caused by modification of gene expression rather than by an alteration of the genetic code itself. That might not tell us very much but it really is an important statement! It's no longer simply a case of identifying which particular genes you have. We now know that it's the way your genes are influenced and made to work that makes the difference. Gene expression accounts for so many of our characteristics. And changes in gene expression have been related to a very wide range of environmental influences and that includes – are you ready for this? – what we eat! Yes, that's absolutely right. The kind of food we consume every single day, the quality of the food we eat, the eating choices we make all contribute far more to our total health and well being than was ever appreciated before. It's not a question of being pre-programmed by our DNA. We've been bombarded by articles and news items for decades telling us every day that everything in our lives is caused by our genes. But what if it isn't just the genetic luck of the draw? What if our health is connected far more to how we live, to what we eat and a whole range of external factors that we can influence? What if we're not programmed to be fat? What if it's about the choices we make? It's becoming increasingly clear that the choices we make are incredibly important to our health and well being. This means we really can influence our health right now right down to the cellular level and that obviously includes our weight as well. This is the breakthrough in our understanding that is revolutionising our entire approach to health and weight control. Our genes do not determine our weight. The answer is not in your genetic code. It's on the end of your fork!

So when we consult the latest reference works in this exciting new area of scientific research, we find that Epigenetics demonstrates the importance of influences which are firmly outside the traditional genetic system. This is the conclusion of Lyle Armstrong, whose research programme is widely respected at the Institute of Genetic Medicine at Newcastle University in the United Kingdom.

Modern biology is rewriting our understanding of genetics, disease and inherited characteristics. This is the view of Nessa Carey in her fascinating book "The Epigenetics Revolution".

Diet is a much easier subject to study than stress or other behaviours. It's been much easier to explore the effects of diet on epigenetics than the effects of the wider environment. So we know a great deal about the way food impacts on our genes. The way we digest food involves the extraction and processing of nutrients that enter specific metabolic pathways. One of these metabolic pathways is responsible for producing the methyl groups and it is these methyl molecules that are highly significant in influencing gene expression in our DNA. So what should we take to encourage this important methyl-producing pathway? Folic acid, the B vitamins and SAM-e (S-Adenosyl Methionine) are essential components for encouraging healthy production levels of the methyl. Diets that are rich in these nutrients can have a rapid and dramatic effect on gene expression.

Intelligent nutrition and appropriate exercise promote efficient fat-burning, healthy muscle building, longevity and wellness. Using your body's natural ability to respond to good nutrition, we can turn away forever from the nightmare of gaining and storing fat, losing muscle mass. We can reduce the risk of disease and illness. A brighter future beckons. The promise of Epigenetics.

As we mentioned before, our physical characteristics are largely based on our parents' DNA. Protecting your DNA from malfunction is not a luxury option anymore. It's an essential task for all of us to undertake to ensure better health, quality of life and sustainable wellbeing. Dr Trygve Tollefsbol wrote in the 2010 edition of Clinical Epigenetics that adding methyl-modifying compounds to the diet can help reduce the incidence and severity of disease. So we know from all the evidence that is being produced on a daily basis that you can reprogram your genes to favour weight loss, improve overall health and boost longevity by following three very simple procedures. You might want to put these ideas on your fridge right now!

Summary - Epigenetics

Your genetic profile is not the full story

Your genes can be switched on and off

The food you eat is the key to influencing your genetic responses

Methylation and diet change the rules of the genetic game

Managing insulin levels by eliminating all grains

Eat Lean, Clean and Good fats

Take practical steps to address food addiction

Chapter 4

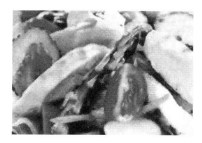

The Paleo Diet (the Epigenetic Way)

Welcome to Your brand new and exciting career! You are now Managing Director of Your Epigenetic Eating Life. Inc. Congratulations. It's simply the Best Job in the Whole World and now it's yours.

Your most important job from now on is to focus on making the right food choices. You don't need to weigh or measure, you don't need to count calories. Wow, I bet that sounds like a new way of dealing with the old weight loss issue, doesn't it? Just make that one decision to follow the programme under any and all circumstances, under any amount of stress and your body will do the rest.

Your only job?

The most important job in your life!

Eat The Right Paleo Food for Your Epigenetic Expression

Fall madly in love with your absolute best weight-loss foods - and watch them fall in love with you and your new, skinnier body

From all the information you've absorbed so far, you'll know for sure that certain food groups (like sugars, grains and dairy products) could be having a very negative impact on your health and wellbeing without you even noticing. But when you think about your present state of wellbeing, you might be wondering how much of your health - or lack of it - has been caused by the food you've been eating. Weight loss is a great example. If you've tried to lose weight but always found it a struggle, experiencing initial success but then putting the pounds back on, you know that you have to do something different. It's time to recognise that cutting down the calories isn't enough. If you're still eating the wrong foods, the problems will remain. It's time to remove the source of the problem and that's only going to happen by removing all the harmful, toxic foods from your diet.

Say goodbye to all the psychologically unhealthy, hormone-unbalancing, gut-disrupting, inflammatory food groups and see the weight fall off. That's right. You might want to read that sentence again. It's essential to your future health. Let your body heal and recover from the years and years of weight gain and from all the other nasty effects of those nasty, toxic foods. It's time to re-programme your metabolism and flush away the inflammation.

Learn once and for all how the foods you've been eating are really affecting your health, your weight and your long term health. We've arrived at one of the most important reasons for you to follow this programme.

This is about to change your life.

Epigenetics demonstrates the vital link between the things you do and how you live to the way your body behaves, all the way down to the cellular level. This might be one of the most surprising revelations about the entire body transformation programme. I think you're going to like it because you're going to love the results.

We cannot possibly put enough emphasis on this simple fact.

Like many of the most important elements in our lives, the answers are so simple that it's too easy to blink and miss the power of this revelation.

The Paleo Eating Transformation

Are you ready for this?

Well, take a deep breath, my friend, because this is the answer you've been waiting for.

Eat. Real. Food.

Eat real food.

Only eat real food.

And now you know.

Real food is unprocessed, additive free and as natural as nature intended.

Real food includes lean, organic game and poultry, line caught seafood, organic free range eggs, tons of fresh vegetables, some fruit, and plenty of good fats from fruits, oils, nuts and seeds.

Eat foods with very few ingredients and no additives, chemicals, sugars or flavourings. Better yet, eat foods with no ingredients listed at all because then they're totally natural and unprocessed.

Don't worry, these guidelines are outlined in extensive detail in our essential life-enhancing Epigenetic Eating Shopping list. Get more Info here www.skinnydeliciouslife.com

Limitation Foods – be careful 5%

High sugar fruits – watermelon, grapes, mangoes.

Buckwheat and quinoa – it behaves like a starchy carbohydrate a bit

Clever but slightly naughty indulgences – 10%

Chocolate – organic cocoa powder,

 Fried potatoes – use sweet potatoes or lots of vinegar to help with digestion,

Muffins cakes and cookies with almond and coconut flour and stevia

Nut and Seed Butters..its ok but still processed

Fats to help you burn fat – 20--%

Coconut oil, extra virgin olive oil, walnuts, macadamias and their oils, coconut products, avocados

Vegetables to fuel your system 30%

Really go to town and enjoy as many servings in as many formats as you can...raw is best, but steamed and stir fried work wonderfully well

Proteins for weight loss 35%

Fish, Turkey (chicken if you must), game and hemp seed protein are the best forms for weight loss

Click Here to Download Your Free Paleo Epigenetic Shopping Guide

www.beranparry.com

Chapter 5

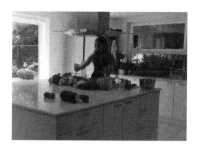

365 PALEO (Epigenetic) Recipes

NO GRAIN BREAKFAST

1. Gutsy Granola
2. Spicy Granola
3. High Protein Breakfast Gold
4. Apple Breakfast Dream
5. Divine Protein Muesli
6. Ultimate Skinny Granola
7. Apple Chia Delight
8. Tasty Apple Almond Coconut Medley
9. Choco Nut Skinny Muesli Balls
10. Sweetie Skinny Crackers

EGGIE MEALS

11. Scrambled Eggs with Chilli
12. Basil and Walnut Eggs Divine
13. Spicy Scrambled Eggs
14. Spicy India Omelet
15. Spectacular Spinach Omelet
16. Blushing Blueberry Omelet
17. Mediterranean Supercharger Omelet with Fennel and Dill
18. Outstanding Veggie Omelet

47. Moroccan Madness

48. Golden Glazed Drumsticks

49. Spicy Grilled Turkey Recipe

50. Piquant Peanut Chicken

51. Cheeky Chicken Salad

52. Melting Mustard Chicken

53. Tantalizing Turkey with Roasted Vegetables

54. Grilled Ostrich Steak

55. Lemony Chicken and Asparagus

56. Delish Chicken Soup

57. Chicken Paprika Surprise

58. Chicken Healing Soup

59. Chicken a la King

60. Chicken Coconut Divine

61. Skinny Turkey Lettuce Fajitas

62. Chicken Jerez

63. Leeky Chicken

64. Zesty Chicken Lemon

65. Sweety Chicky Soup

66. Chicken Zoodle Delish

67. Coconut Turkey Salad

68. Creamy Chicken Mushroom Soup Bonanza

69. Feisty Filipino Chicken

70. Chinese Chicken Legs

71. Jolly Jamaican Chicken

72. Citrus Chicken

73. Beautiful Baked Chicken

74. South American Chicken

75. Rosemary Chicken

76. Sexy Sesame Turkey

77. Pollo Al Vinagre

78. Chicken Caully Delish

79. Courgette Spaghetti with Delish Chicken

80. Chicken Pea Stir Fry

81. Chicken Pineapple Delight

82. Chicken Peanut Lettuce Wraps

MAIN COURSE - FISH

83. Thai Baked Fish with Squash Noodles

84. Divine Prawn Mexicana

85. Superior Salmon with Lemon and Thyme OR Use any White fish

86. Spectacular Shrimp Scampi in Spaghetti Sauce

87. Scrumptious Cod in Delish Sauce

88. Delish Baked dill Salmon

89. Prawn garlic Fried "Rice"

90. Lemon and Thyme Super Salmon

91. Delicious Salmon in Herb Crust

92. Salmon Mustard Delish

93. Sexy Spicy Salmon

94. Mouthwatering Stuffed Salmon

95. Spectacular Salmon

96. Creamy Coconut Salmon

97. Salmon Dill Bonanza

98. Sexy Shrimp Cocktail

99. Gambas al Ajillo--Sizzling Garlic Shrimp

100. Garlic Lemon Shrimp Bonanza

101. Courgette Pesto and Shrimp

102. Easy Shrimp Stir Fry

103. Delectable Shrimp Scampi

104. Citrus Shrimp Delux
105. Sexy Garlic Shrimp
106. Shrimp Cakes Delux
107. Shrimp Spinach Spectacular
108. Prawn Salad Boats
109. Cheeky Curry Shrimp
110. Courgette Shrimp Coquettes
111. Sexy Shrimp on Sticks
112. Delicious Fish Stir Fry
113. Sexy Shrimp with Delish Veggie Stir Fry
114. Sexy Spicy Salmon
115. Delish Skewered Shrimp
116. Lemon Tilapia Ajillo
117. Tantalizing Prawn Skewers
118. Seared Salmon with Mango Salsa
119. Sexy Rosemary Salmon
120. Broiled Curry Coconut Sole or Cod
121. Oregano Prawns
122. Tasty Tomato Tilapia
123. Prawn Asparagus Stir Fry
124. Cilantro Fish Delish
125. Perfect Prawns
126. Fish Fillet Delux
127. Gambas Ajillo
128. Peachy Prawn Coconut
129. Highly Delish Herb Salmon
130. Happy Halibut Soup
131. Tasty Teriyaki Salmon
132. Sexy Shrimp Cakes

161. Chinese Divine Salad

162. Divinely Delish Salad Surprise

163. Avocado Salad with Cilantro and Lime

164. Mexican Medley Salad

165. Macadamia Nut Chicken/Turkey Salad

166. Red Cabbage Bonanza Salad

167. Spectacular Sprouts Salad

168. Avocado Egg Salad

169. Avocado Divine Salad

170. Classic Waldorf Salad

171. Artichoke Heart & Turkey Salad Radicchio Cups

172. Tempting Tuna Stuffed Tomato

173. Incredibly Delish Avocado Tuna Salad

174. Italian Tuna Bonanza Salad

175. Asian Aspiration Salad

176. Tasty Carrot Salad

177. Creamy Carrot Salad

178. Sublime Courgette Tomato Salad

179. Brussels Muscles Sprouts

180. Blushing Beet Salad

181. Sashimi Divine with Vinaigrette

182. Grilled Shrimp Fennel Salad

183. Chicken Delish Salad

184. Sea Scallops Sensation

PURE VEGETABLES

185. Vegetarian Curry with Squash

186. Saucy Gratin with Creamy Cauliflower Bonanza

187. Egg Bok Choy and Basil Stir-Fry

188. Skinny Eggie Vegetable Stir Fry

273. Divine Butternut Chips
274. Outstanding Orange Skinny Snack
275. Spicy Pumpkin Seed Bonanza
276. Delectable Chocolate-Frosted Doughnuts
277. Eggplant Divine
278. Choco Apple Nachos
279. Skinny Delicious Snack Bars
280. Pumpkin Vanilla Delight
281. Skinny Quicky Crackers
282. Delectable Parsnip Chips
283. Spicy Crunchy Skinny Snack
284. Raw Hemp Kale Bars
285. Skinny Trail Mix
286. Anti-Aging Fruit Delights
287. Paleo Rosemary Sweet Potato Crunches
288. Apple Peach Skinny Bars
289. Spicy Fried Almonds
290. Zucchini Avocado Hummus
291. Skinny Power Snack
292. Skinny Salsa
293. Divine Turkey Stuffed Tomatoes
294. Curried Nutty Delish
295. Skinny Chips
296. Zesty Zucchini Pesto Roll-ups
297. Butternut Squash-raw Veggie Dip
298. Skinny Power Balls
299. Chocolate Goji SKinny Bars
300. Delish Cashew Butter Treats
301. Skinny Veggie Dip

SOUP

302. Roasted Tasty Tomato Soup

303. Thai Coconut Turkey Soup

304. Cheeky Chicken Soup

305. Triple Squash Delight Soup

306. Ginger Carrot Delight Soup

307. Wonderful Watercress Soup

308. Curried Butternut Soup

309. Celery Cashew Cream Soup

310. Mighty Andalusian Gazpacho

311. Munchy Mushroom Soup

312. Tempting Tomato Basil Soup

313. Healing Chicken/Turkey Vegetable Soup

314. Sumptuous Saffron Turkey Cauliflower Soup

315. Delicious Masala Soup

316. Creamy Chicken Soup

317. Delicious Lemon-Garlic Soup

318. Turkey Squash Soup

319. Roasted Winter Vegetable Turkey Soup

320. Zucchini Fish Soup Delight!

321. Cheeky Cabbage Soup

322. Bold Butternut Soup

323. Espana Gazpacho Salmorejo

324. Kale Turkey Delight

325. Turkey Zuccini Soup

326. Tantalizing Turkey Meatball Soup

327. Divine Acorn Squash Soup

328. Piquant Pumpkin Soup

329. Tomato Turkey Bisque

BEVERAGES

330. Wonderful Watermelon water

331. Chia Peach Fresca

332. Divine Ice Tea with Fresh Mint

333. Raspberry Bellini

334. Pomegranate Peach Vodka

335. Devillish Margarita

336. Melon Martinis

STARTERS

337. Tasty Testy Lettuce Wraparounds

338. Sexy Venison or Steak Skewers

339. Avocado and Tuna Surprise

340. Avocado and Peach Salsa

341. Baked Crispy Sweet Potato Fries

342. Baked Salmon or Tuna Cakes with Red Pepper Chipotle Lime Sauce

343. Baked Prawn Cakes

344. Delish Fries with Garlic Aioli

345. Baked Divine Plantains

346. Sexy Turkey Croquettes

347. Stunning Zesty Shrimp

348. Avocado, Cucumber and Tomato Salad

349. Sashimi Cucumber Cups

350. Divine Calamari Lemon Salad Surprise

351. Incredible Lobster Salad

352. Turkey and Zucchini Yakitori

353. Grilled Gorgeous Prawn Kebabs

354. Great Guacamole

355. Pumpkin Avocado Salad

356. Titillating Turkey Kebabs

Chapter 6

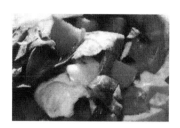

365 Paleo Epigenetic Recipes

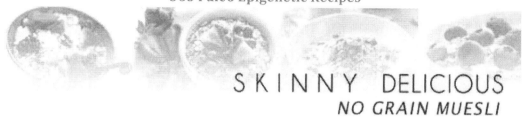

NO GRAIN BREAKFAST

1. Gutsy Granola
Ingredients:

1 cup cashews

3/4 cup almonds

1/4 cup pumpkin seeds, shelled

1/4 cup sunflower seeds, shelled

1/2 cup unsweetened coconut flakes

1/4 cup coconut oil

Stevia to taste

1 tsp vanilla

1 tsp low sodium salt

Instructions:

Preheat oven to 300 degrees F. Line a baking sheet with parchment paper. Place the cashews, almonds, coconut flakes and pumpkin seeds into a blender and pulse to break the mixture into smaller pieces.

In a large microwave-safe bowl, melt the coconut oil, vanilla, and stevia together for 40-50 seconds. Add in the mixture from the blender and the sunflower seeds, and stir to coat.

Spread the mixture out onto the baking sheet and cook for 20-25 minutes, stirring once, until the mixture is lightly browned. Remove from heat. Add low sodium salt.

Press the granola mixture together to form a flat, even surface. Cool for about 15 minutes, and then break into chunks.

2. Spicy Granola

Ingredients:

1 ½ cups almond flour

1/3 cup coconut oil

2 tsp cinnamon

2 tsp nutmeg

2 tsp vanilla extract

½ cup walnuts

½ cup coconut flakes

¼ cup hemp seeds

low sodium salt, to taste

Instructions:

Preheat oven to 275 degrees Fahrenheit.

Combine all ingredients in a large mixing bowl and mix well. (I find it easier to melt down the coconut oil a little bit before adding it)

Spread mixture into one flat layer on a greased baking sheet.

Bake for 40-50 minutes, or until mixture is toasted to your liking.

Remove from oven and allow to cool before serving, then transfer into a plastic container to save the rest!

3. High Protein Breakfast Gold

Ingredients:

1/2 c. Flax-Meal, golden

1/2 c. Chia seed

Stevia liquid to taste

2 tbs. dark ground cinnamon

1 tbs. hemp protein powder

2 tbs. coconut oil, melted

1 tsp. vanilla extract
3/4 c. + 2 tbs. hot water

Instructions:

Begin to spread the dough out until its super thin, onto a parchment paper lined cookie sheet. Bake at 325 for 15 minutes, then drop it down to 300 and leave for 30 minutes. Before dropping it, pull out the sheet and cut it using a pizza roller.

Put it back into the oven exactly like this, don't separate the pieces. When the 30 minutes are up, pull it out and separate the pieces. Drop the pieces to 200 degrees F for 1 hour. They will be completely dried out at this point. Enjoy with almond milk!

4. Apple Breakfast Dream

Ingredients:

2 C raw walnuts

1 C raw macadamia nuts

2 apples, peeled and diced

1 Tbsp coconut oil

1 Tbsp ground cinnamon

2 C almond milk

1 14 oz can full fat coconut milk

Instructions:

Combine nuts and dates in a food processor until ground into a fine meal, about 1 minute; set aside.

Saute apples over medium heat in coconut oil until lightly browned, about 5 minutes.

Add nut mixture and cinnamon to apples and stir to incorporate, about 1 minute.

Reduce heat to low and add coconut and almond milk.

Stirring occasionally, let mixture cook uncovered until thickened, about 25 minutes.

5. Divine Protein Muesli

Ingredients:

1 cup unsweetened unsulfured coconut flakes

1 tbsp chopped walnuts

1 tbsp raw almonds (~10)

1 tbsp chocolate chips (soy, dairy, and gluten free brand)

1/2 tsp cinnamon (Ceylon)

1 cup unsweetened almond milk

1 scoop hemp protein

Instructions:

In a medium bowl layer coconut flakes, walnuts, almonds, raisins and chocolate chips.

Sprinkle with cinnamon.

Pour cold almond milk over the muesli and eat with a spoon.

6. Ultimate Skinny Granola

Ingredients:

1 cup of unsweetened coconut milk or unsweetened almond milk or kefir

Stevia liquid to taste

1 tspoon of unsalted pecan pieces

1 tspoon of unsalted walnut pieces

1 tspoon of silvered almonds

1 tspoon of unsalted pistachios

1 tspoon of unsalted raw pine nuts

1 tspoon of unsalted, raw sunflower/safflower seeds

1 tspoon of unsalted, raw pumpkin seeds

2 Tbspoons of frozen or fresh berry selection (e.g. blueberries, blackberries, raspberries, strawberries, or other kinds etc)

Instructions:

Put all the nuts & seeds in a breakfast bowl.

If using unsweetened milk, you could optionally add a teaspoon of pure liquid stevia and stir it well in.

Add the berries and milk.

If using frozen berries, wait for 2-3 minutes for them to get warmer.

The berries will now release some color into the milk, making it look really interesting. Enjoy!

7. Apple Chia Delight

Ingredients:

2c organic chia seeds (black or white)

1c organic hemp hearts

1/2 chopped dried organic apples (or other dried fruit of your choice)

2tbsp real cinnamon

1 tsp low sodium salt

optional: 1/2c chopped nuts of your choice

Instructions:

Throw all of this together, mix it up, and store in a jar in a cool dry place. Stevia to taste.

8. Tasty Apple Almond Coconut Medley
Ingredients:

one-half apple cored and roughly diced

handful of sliced almonds

handful of unsweetened coconut

generous dose of cinnamon

1 pinch of low sodium salt

Instructions:

Pulse in the food processor to desired consistency—smaller is better for the little ones! Serve with almond milk, or creamy coconut milk.

9. Choco Nut Skinny Muesli Balls
Ingredients:

1 cup of raw almonds

1 Tablespoon of coconut oil

¼ teaspoon low sodium salt

2 Tablespoon Coconut flour

1 egg white

2 Tablespoon plus 1 teaspoon of Cacao powder

¼ cup of pure liquid stevia

Instructions:

First grind the almonds in a food processor or blender until you have a flour.

Add the ground almonds, low sodium salt, coconut flour, egg white, pure liquid stevia and cacao power to a bowl and mix with a spoon until you have a dough.

Either:

a) Place the dough onto a piece of parchment paper. Place a second piece of parchment paper over the top and roll it until it is ¼" thick. With a wet knife, score it into 1" squares. Place the parchment paper on a baking sheet when finished.

Or

b) Take a small pinch of the dough and roll into a ¼ round ball and set on a baking sheet lined with parchment paper.

Turn on your oven and set to 350 degrees and bake for 15 - 18 minutes for cereal balls or bake for 8 to 12 minutes for flat cereal.

Remove from the oven and let cool on the pan.

Top with your favorite milk and enjoy!

10. Sweetie Skinny Crackers
Ingredients:

1 egg

pure liquid stevia to taste

1 Tbspn coconut oil, melted

1.5 cups almond flour

5 cup coconut flour

1 teaspoon cinnamon

Instructions:

Preheat oven to 350°

In a large bowl, whisk together the egg, pure liquid stevia and melted coconut oil

Add the coconut and almond flour and stir to combine.

Give the dough a couple of kneads so it's well incorporated.

Turn the dough onto a piece of parchment paper and flatten a bit with your hands.

Place another piece of parchment on top and roll out with a rolling pin until it's about 1/8 inch thick.

Remove the top piece of parchment and cut the dough into 1/4 inch squares for cereal, and about 2"x3" for crackers

Sprinkle the cinnamon into the dough mixture.

Slide the dough with the bottom parchment paper onto a baking sheet and bake for 15 minutes.

Turn down the oven to 325° and bake for another 10-15 minutes, or until the cereal / crackers are crisp.

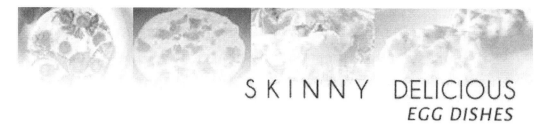

SKINNY DELICIOUS
EGG DISHES

EGGIE MEALS

11. Scrambled Eggs with Chilli
Ingredients:

4 fresh green chillies with skins removed

2 tablespoons (30g or 1 oz) coconut oil

1 small onion, peeled and finely chopped

6 eggs

1/4 cup (62ml or 2 fl oz) coconut milk

1/4 teaspoon (1ml) low sodium salt

Instructions:

After removing chilli skins, remove and discard seeds and finely chop remaining chilli.

Beat eggs, coconut milk and salt in a bowl and set aside.

Heat oil in a medium size saucepan over a medium heat.

Reduce heat to low and add egg mixture to saucepan and mix well.

Scatter chillies over mixture.

Cook over a low heat until eggs are cooked.

Serves 4. Serve hot.

12. Basil and Walnut Eggs Divine
Ingredients:

3 organic eggs

1/2 cup fresh basil, chopped

1/3 cup walnuts, chopped

salt and pepper

Instructions:

Whisk eggs in a bowl then place in a frying pan on medium heat, stirring constantly.

When the eggs are almost cooked, add the basil and continue cooking for a further 1 minute or until eggs are fully cooked.

Add salt and pepper to taste.

Remove from heat and stir in the walnuts before serving.

13. Spicy Scrambled Eggs

Ingredients:

1 tablespoon extra virgin olive oil

1 red onion, finely chopped

1 medium green pepper, cored, seeded, and finely chopped

1 chile, seeded and cut into thin strips

3 ripe tomatoes, peeled, seeded, and chopped

Salt and freshly ground black pepper

4 large organic eggs

Instructions:

Heat the olive oil in a large, heavy, preferably nonstick skillet over medium heat.

Add the onion and cook until soft, 6 to 7 minutes.

Add the pepper and chile and continue cooking until soft, another 4 to 5 minutes.

Add in the tomatoes, and salt and pepper to taste and cook uncovered, over low heat for 10 minutes.

Add the eggs, stirring them into the mixture to distribute.

Cover the skillet and cook until the eggs are set but still fluffy and tender, about 7 to 8 minutes. Divide between 4 plates and serve.

14. Spicy India Omelet

Ingredients:

3 Eggs

1 Onion, chopped

4 Green Chilli (optional)

1/4 cup Coconut grated

Low sodium Salt, Oil - as required

Instructions:

Beat the Eggs severely.

Mix chopped onion, rounded green chilli, salt and grated coconuts with eggs.

Heat oil on a medium-low heat, in a pan.

Pour the mixture in the form of pancakes and cook it on the both sides.

15. Spectacular Spinach Omelet

Ingredients:

2 eggs

1.5 cups raw spinach

coconut oil, about 1 tbsp

1/3 c tomatoes and onion salsa (lightly fried in pan)

1 tbsp fresh cilantro

Instructions:

Melt coconut oil on medium in frying pan. Add spinach, cook until mostly wilted. Beat eggs and add to pan.

Flip once the egg sets around the edge. When it's almost done add the salsa on top just to warm it. Move to plate and add cilantro. Serves one.

16. Blushing Blueberry Omelet

Ingredients:

2 eggs

1 tsp. vanilla extract

coconut oil

1/2 c. blueberries

Stevia to taste

Instructions:

Lightly beat two eggs and vanilla extract in a bowl. Heat 6" non-stick pan over medium heat.

While pan is heating, heat half the blueberries in a saucepan until juices flow.

Add coconut oil to non-stick pan and coat evenly.

When thoroughly heated, add egg mixture. Swish once and let sit.

When eggs are about 70% settled, swish again. There should be a nice crispy layer around the side of the pan.

When it starts to separate from the side, add fresh and cooked blueberries to omelet, reserving a few for garnish.

Crispy layer should really be pulling away from pan now.

Use a fork to help fold the omelet over. Slide on to plate, top with reserved blueberry filling, and enjoy

17. Mediterranean Supercharger Omelet with Fennel and Dill

Ingredients:

2 tablespoons olive oil, divided

2 cups thinly sliced fresh fennel bulb, fronds chopped and reserved

8 cherry tomatoes

5 large eggs, beaten to blend with 1/4 teaspoon salt and 1/4 teaspoon ground black pepper

1 1/2 tablespoons chopped fresh dill

Instructions:

Add remaining 1 tablespoon oil to same skillet; heat over medium-high heat.

Add beaten eggs and cook until eggs are just set in center, tilting skillet and lifting edges of omelet with spatula to let uncooked portion flow underneath, about 3 minutes.

Top with fennel mixture. Sprinkle dill over.

Using spatula, fold uncovered half of omelet over; slide onto plate.

Garnish with chopped fennel and serve.

18. Outstanding Veggie Omelet

Ingredients:

3 eggs, beaten

1 carrot, matchstick cut

3 scallions, diagonal sliced

1 handful tiny broccoli florets or whatever leftover veggies you have

Bits of leftover cooked turkey

Safflower oil

Low sodium salt

Instructions:

Heat oil in a wok or large cast iron skillet over medium heat, until hot enough to sizzle a drop of water.

Add broccoli and carrots, stir fry 2 min. until soft.

Add cooked turkey, stir fry 1 min. until heated through. Add scallions and eggs, scramble. Add salt to taste. Serve.

19. Spicy Spinach Bake

Ingredients:

6 eggs

1 bunch fresh spinach chopped (a box of frozen will do if you do not have fresh)

1/2 tsp hot pepper flakes

Olive oil

Low sodium Salt and pepper

Instructions:

Scramble the eggs in a bowl. Add the spinach, low sodium salt and pepper.

Scramble together. Heat a large non-stick skillet with about 1/2 cup olive oil.

When the oil is hot put the hot pepper flakes in then pour the mixture in. When it starts to cook on the bottom, flip it over.

Try not to cook it until it is dry, take it out when it is medium scrambled. Let cool and eat.

20. Delish Veggie Hash With Eggs

Ingredients:

2 tablespoon extra virgin olive oil

2 garlic cloves, minced

1/4 cup sweet white onion, chopped

1 cup yellow squash, chopped

1/2 cup mushroom, sliced

Low sodium salt and pepper

1 cup cherry tomatoes, halved

1 cup fresh spinach, chopped

4 eggs, poached or cooked any style

You can substitute the squash with whatever vegetables you have

Instructions:

Heat large non-stick skillet over medium heat. Add olive oil to pan.

Add garlic and onion and saute for 2 minutes, then add chopped squash or your favorite vegetable, cook for 2 more minutes, then add mushrooms. Cook for 5-minutes or until almost compete.

At this point add low sodium salt and pepper, then add tomatoes and spinach and cook until spinach wilts. Drain well before plating.

While finishing this prepare eggs to your liking in another pan.

To serve, drained hash mixture to and then add to individual plates. On top of hash add 2 cooked eggs per person.

21. Spectacular Eggie Salsa

Ingredients:

2 pounds fresh ripe tomatoes, peeled and coarsely chopped

2 to 3 serrano or jalapeño chiles, seeded for a milder sauce, and chopped

2 garlic cloves, peeled, halved, green shoots removed

1/2 small onion, chopped

2 tablespoons oil

Low sodium salt to taste

4 to 8 eggs (to taste)

Chopped cilantro for garnish

Instructions:

Place the tomatoes, chiles, garlic and onion in a blender and puree, retaining a bit of texture.

Heat 1 tablespoon of the oil over high heat in a large, heavy nonstick skillet, until a drop of puree will sizzle when it hits the pan.

Add the puree and cook, stirring, for four to ten minutes, until the sauce thickens, darkens and leaves a trough when you run a spoon down the middle of the pan. It should just begin to stick to the pan.

Season to taste with salt, and remove from the heat. Keep warm while you fry the eggs.

Warm four plates. Fry the eggs in a heavy skillet over medium-high heat.

Use the remaining tablespoon of oil if necessary. Cook them sunny side up, until the whites are solid but the yolks still runny.

Season with salt and pepper, and turn off the heat. Place one or two fried eggs on each plate.

Spoon the hot salsa over the whites of the eggs, leaving the yolks exposed if possible. Sprinkle with cilantro and serve.

22. Mushrooms, Eggs and Onion Bonanza
Ingredients:

1 medium onion, finely diced

1/4 cup coconut oil

10-12 medium white mushrooms, finely chopped

12 hard boiled eggs, peeled and finely chopped

Freshly ground black pepper to taste

Instructions:

Saute the onion in coconut oil until golden brown.

Add the mushrooms and saute another 5 minutes or so, stirring frequently, until mushrooms are softened and turned dark.

Remove from heat and let cool.

Mix together with the eggs and pepper. Chill until ready to serve.

23. Avocado and Shrimp Omelet
Ingredients:

6 eggs

2 Tbsp. chopped parsley

2 Tbsp. lemon juice, divided

1/4 tsp. salt

1/8 tsp. cayenne pepper

1 large* ripe avocado, diced

1 1/2 Tbsp. avocado oil

3 oz. bay shrimp

3 parsley sprigs

Instructions:

Beat together eggs, parsley, 3/4 of the lemon juice, salt, and cayenne pepper; reserve.

Gently toss avocado with remaining lemon juice; reserve.

Heat oil in an omelet pan. (Use a large omelet pan for four or more servings.)

Pour egg mixture into pan.

Cook over medium heat, lifting edges and tilting pan to allow uncooked egg to run under, until set but still moist on top.

Scatter reserved avocado and shrimp over omelet.

Fold omelet in half; heat another minute or two.

Slide onto a warmed serving plate; garnish with parsley sprigs.

To serve, cut omelet into wedges.

24. Delish Veggie Breakfast Peppers

Ingredients:

2 bell peppers – your choice of color

4 eggs

1 cup white mushrooms

1 cup broccoli

¼ tsp cayenne pepper

low sodium salt and pepper, to taste

Instructions:

Preheat oven to 375 degrees Fahrenheit.

Dice up your vegetables of choice.

In a medium sized bowl, mix eggs, low sodium salt, pepper, cayenne pepper, and vegetables.

Cut peppers into equal halves. A tip:

Core the peppers so that they're clean enough to add the filling.

Pour a quarter of the egg / vegetable mix into each pepper halve, adding more vegetables to the top to fill in any empty space.

Place on baking sheet and cook approximately 35 minutes.

25. Breakfast Mexicana
Ingredients:

For the tortillas:

2 eggs

2 egg whites

1/2 cup water

4 tsp ground flaxseed

Pinch of low sodium salt

For the filling:

1 avocado, diced

1/4 cup red bell

pepper, finely diced

1/4 cup onion, finely diced

1/4 cup baked cod or other protein

Handful of spinach leaves

1 tsp coconut oil

Instructions:

In a small bowl, whisk together the ingredients for the tortilla. Preheat the oven

Heat a 10-inch non-stick skillet over medium heat and coat well with coconut oil spray.

Pour half of the tortilla mixture into the pan and swirl to evenly distribute.

Using a metal spatula, loosen the edges of the tortilla from the pan.

Cook a couple of minutes until golden brown on the bottom, and then carefully slide the spatula under the tortilla to loosen it from the bottom of the pan. Do not flip yet.

Place the pan under the broiler for 3-4 minutes until the tortilla gets a little bubbly.

Remove the tortilla from the pan, setting on a piece of aluminum foil. Repeat with other half of tortilla mixture.

After the tortillas are done broiling, preheat the oven to 400 degrees F. In a separate small pan, heat the coconut oil over medium heat.

Add the onions and peppers and sauté for 5-8 minutes, until soft. Add the spinach into the pan and wilt.

Place all of the fillings down the center of the tortillas and wrap tightly. Place into the oven for 5-8 minutes to set. It's so delish!

26. Zucchini Casserole

Ingredients:

3 large zucchini

1/2 red onion, chopped

1/2 cup mushrooms

5 eggs

1 tsp low sodium salt

Freshly ground black pepper, to taste

Instructions:

Preheat oven to 375 degrees F..

Grate all of the zucchini and put into a large bowl.

In a separate bowl, beat the eggs with low sodium salt and pepper.

Combine all of the ingredients, in the large bowl and mix together. You want to have enough eggs to coat the whole mixture.

Warm about a 1/2 tablespoon of olive oil in the skillet over medium heat.

Add the zucchini mixture into the pan. Cover and cook about 5 minutes until the eggs start to set on the bottom.

Transfer to the oven and bake for 12-15 minutes, until the eggs are firm. Remove and let rest for 5-10 minutes, then serve.

27. Blueberry Nut Casserole

Ingredients:

Crush one cup almonds, walnuts and pecans with one teaspoon olive oil and bake in the oven at 200 for 20 minutes

2 cups frozen blueberries

5 eggs

1 cup almond milk

Stevia to taste

1 tsp vanilla extract

1 tsp cinnamon

Pinch of nutmeg

Instructions:

Preheat the oven to 350 degrees F. Grease an 8x8-inch baking dish with coconut oil spray. Place the nut crust and blueberries into the dish.

Whisk together the eggs, almond milk, stevia, vanilla, and cinnamon in a medium bowl.

Pour the egg mixture over the crust and blueberries. Lightly stir to coat.

Bake for 35-45 minutes. Remove from the oven and allow the casserole to rest for 15 minutes before serving.

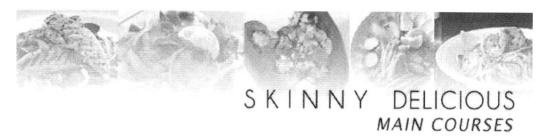

SKINNY DELICIOUS
MAIN COURSES

MAIN COURSE - CHICKEN

28. Spicy Turkey Stir Fry

Ingredients:

2 lbs. boneless skinless chicken or turkey breasts, cut into 1-inch slices

2 tbsp coconut oil

1 tsp cumin seeds

1/2 each green, red, and orange bell pepper, thinly sliced

1 tsp garam masala

2 tsp freshly ground pepper

low sodium salt, to taste

Scallions, for garnish

For the marinade:

1/2 cup coconut cream

1 clove garlic, minced

1 tsp ginger, minced

1 tbsp freshly ground pepper

2 tsp low sodium salt

1/4 tsp turmeric

Instructions:

Place all of the marinade ingredients into a Ziploc bag. Add the chicken, close the bag, and shake to coat.

Marinate in the refrigerator for at least 30 minutes, or up to 6 hours.

In a wok or large sauté pan, melt the coconut oil over medium-high heat. Add the cumin seeds and cook for 2-3 minutes.

Add the marinated chicken and let cook for 5 minutes. Stir the chicken until it begins to brown, and then add the peppers, garam masala, and freshly ground pepper.

Sprinkle with low sodium salt. Cook for 4-5 minutes, stirring regularly, or until the bell pepper is cooked to desired doneness. Serve hot.

29. Turkey and Kale Pasta Casserole
Ingredients:

1 lb. Turkey breast

1 medium spaghetti squash, halved and seeded

Extra virgin olive oil, for drizzling

1 large bunch of kale, de-stemmed, and chopped

1/2 red onion, sliced thin

1/3 cup chicken broth

1/2 cup coconut milk

1 clove garlic, minced

2 tsp Italian seasoning

low sodium salt and freshly ground pepper, to taste

Instructions:

Preheat the oven to 400 degrees F. Place the squash in the microwave for 3-4 minutes to soften.

Using a sharp knife, cut the squash in half lengthwise. Scoop out the seeds and discard. Place the halves, with the cut side up, on a rimmed baking sheet.

Drizzle with olive oil and sprinkle with low sodium salt and pepper. Roast in the oven for 45-50 minutes, until you can poke the squash easily with a fork.

Let it cool until you can handle it safely. Then scrape the insides with a fork to shred the squash into strands.

Meanwhile, melt the coconut oil in a large oven-safe skillet over medium heat.

Add the turkey breast and brown. Once cooked through, remove to a plate. In the same skillet, add the onion and sauté for 3-4 minutes.

Next add the garlic, Italian seasoning, and kale and cook for 2-3 minutes to slightly wilt the kale.

Pour in the chicken broth and coconut milk and simmer for an additional 2-3 minutes. Remove from heat.

Stir in the cooked turkey. Add the spaghetti squash into the skillet and stir well to combine.

Bake for 15-18 minutes, until the top has slightly browned. Serve hot.

30. Roasted Lemon Herb Chicken

Ingredients:

12 total pieces bone-in chicken thighs and legs

1 medium onion, thinly sliced

1 tbsp dried rosemary

1 tsp dried thyme

1 lemon, sliced thin

1 orange, sliced thin

For the marinade:

5 tbsp extra virgin olive oil

6 cloves garlic, minced

Stevia to taste

Juice of 1 lemon

Juice of 1 orange

1 tbsp Italian seasoning

1 tsp onion powder

Dash of red pepper flakes

low sodium salt and freshly ground pepper, to taste

Instructions:

Whisk together all of the marinade ingredients in a small bowl. Place the chicken in a baking dish (or a large Ziploc bag) and pour the marinade over it. Marinate for 3 hours to overnight.

Preheat the oven to 400 degrees F. Place the chicken in a baking dish and arrange with the onion, orange, and lemon slices.

Sprinkle with thyme, rosemary, low sodium salt and pepper. Cover with aluminum foil and bake for 30 minutes.

Remove the foil, baste the chicken, and bake for another 30 minutes uncovered, until the chicken is cooked through.

31. Basil Turkey with Roasted Tomatoes

Ingredients:

2 turkey breasts

1 cup mushrooms, chopped

1/2 medium onion, chopped

1-2 tbsp extra virgin olive oil

Half cup thinly sliced fresh basil

low sodium salt and pepper, to taste

1 pint cherry tomatoes

Stevia to taste

Fresh parsley, for garnish

Instructions:

Preheat the oven to 400 degrees F. Place the tomatoes on a baking sheet and drizzle with olive oil and stevia. Sprinkle with low sodium salt and pepper and toss to coat evenly. Bake for 15-20 minutes until soft.

While the tomatoes are roasting, heat one tablespoon of olive oil in a large pan over low heat. Add the onions and mushrooms and cook for 10-12 minutes to soften and caramelize, stirring regularly. Clear a space for the chicken.

Season the turkey with low sodium salt and pepper and then place it in the pan. Simmer for 15 minutes or until the chicken is cooked through. Every 5 minutes or so, spoon the sauce in the pan over the turkey.

To assemble, divide the tomatoes between two plates. Place one turkey breast on each and then spoon the onions, mushrooms, and pan drippings over the turkey. Garnish with parsley.

32. Roasted and Filled Tasty Bell Peppers

Ingredients:

5 large bell peppers

1 tbsp coconut oil

1/2 large onion, diced

1 tsp dried oregano

1/2 tsp low sodium salt

1 lb. ground turkey

1 large zucchini, halved and diced

3 tbsp tomato paste

Freshly ground black pepper, to taste

Fresh parsley, for serving

Instructions:

Preheat the oven to 350 degrees F. Coat a small baking dish with coconut oil spray. Bring a large pot of water to a boil. Cut the stems and very top of the peppers off, removing the seeds. Place in boiling water for 4-5 minutes. Remove from the water and drain face-down on a paper towel.

Heat the coconut oil in a large nonstick pan over medium heat. Add in the onion. Sauté for 3-4 minutes until the onion begins to soften. Stir in the ground turkey, oregano, low sodium salt, and pepper and cook until turkey is browned.

Add the zucchini to the skillet as the turkey finishes cooking. Cook everything together until the zucchini is soft, and then drain any juices from the pan.

Remove the pan from heat and stir in the tomato paste. Bake for 15 minutes.

33. Chili-Garlic Ostrich or Venison Skewers
Ingredients:

6 Wooden Skewers, soaked in cold water for 30 minutes

2 Ostrich or Venison, diced

1 tbsp. Olive Oil

1 tsp. Red Chilies, seeds removed & finely chopped

4 Garlic Cloves, minced

6 tbsp. fresh lemon juice

Instructions:

Preheat oven to 350 F or preheat barbeque grill on high heat.

To make sauce, combine the oil, chilies, garlic, and lemon juice in a small bowl. Set aside for a few minutes.

Thread diced meat onto skewers and place on an oven tray lined with baking paper.

Pour chili and garlic sauce over the chicken, coating well.

Bake in the oven for 30-40 minutes or until chicken is cooked. If cooking on a grill, cook chicken for 5-6 minutes on each side.

Eat with any of the delicious salad recipes.

34. Creamy Chicken Casserole
Ingredients:

2 cups cubed cooked chicken

1 1/2 cups cooked butternut squash

1/2 cup coconut cream,

1/4 cup coconut oil, melted

1 heaping cup green peas, fresh or frozen

1 tbsp apple cider vinegar

1/2 tsp low sodium salt

1/2 tsp oregano

1/2 tsp thyme

1 tbsp fresh parsley

Instructions:

In a large bowl, mash the butternut squash. Stir in the coconut cream, oil, vinegar, low sodium salt, oregano, and thyme.

Once everything is combined, add in chicken and peas.

Place the mixture into a large saucepan and cook over medium heat for 5-8 minutes.

Top with fresh parsley and serve warm.

35. Spectacular Spaghetti and Delish Turkey Balls
Ingredients:

1 spaghetti squash

Extra virgin olive oil,

low sodium salt and pepper

1 tsp dried or fresh oregano

For the sauce:

1 lb ground turkey

1 small onion, chopped

4 cloves garlic, minced

1 tbsp coconut oil

1 tomato, chopped

1/2 jar of tomato sauce

1 tbsp Italian seasoning

low sodium salt and pepper to taste

Fresh basil

Instructions:

Preheat oven to 400 degrees F. Using a sharp knife, cut the squash in half lengthwise. Scoop out the seeds and discard.

Place the halves with the cut side up on a rimmed baking sheet. Drizzle with olive oil and season with low sodium salt, pepper, and oregano. Roast the squash in the oven for 40-45 minutes, until you can poke the squash easily with a fork.

Let it cool until you can handle it safely. Then scrape the insides with a fork to shred the squash into strands.

While the spaghetti squash is roasting, melt coconut oil in a large skillet over medium heat.

Add chopped onion and garlic and cook for 4-5 minutes. Add ground turkey and brown the meat, stirring occasionally. Season with low sodium salt and pepper.

Add the chopped tomato, tomato sauce, and Italian seasoning and stir to combine. Simmer on low heat, stirring occasionally, while the spaghetti squash finishes roasting. Serve over spaghetti squash with basil for garnish.

36. Sensational Courgette Pasta and Turkey Bolognaise

Ingredients:

4 medium zucchini

For the sauce:

1 lb ground turkey

1 small onion, chopped

4 cloves garlic, minced

1 tbsp coconut oil

1 tomato, chopped

1/2 jar of tomato sauce

1 tbsp Italian seasoning

low sodium salt and pepper to taste

Fresh basil, for garnish

Instructions:

Use a julienne peeler to slice the zucchini into noodles, stopping when you reach the seeds. Set aside.

If cooking zucchini noodles, simply add to a skillet and sauté over medium heat for 4-5 minutes.

Melt coconut oil in a large skillet over medium heat. Add chopped onion and garlic and cook for 4-5 minutes.

Add ground turkey and brown the meat, stirring occasionally. Season with low sodium salt and pepper.

Add the chopped tomato, tomato sauce, and Italian seasoning and stir to combine. Simmer on low heat, stirring occasionally.

Add the sauce to the noodles and ENJOY.

37. Tempting Turkey Spaghetti Squash Boats

Ingredients:

1 medium spaghetti squash or 2 small spaghetti squash

1 1/2 lbs. Turkey mashed

1 yellow onion, diced

4 cloves garlic, minced

1 bunch kale

3 tbsp extra virgin olive oil, plus more for drizzling

low sodium salt and pepper

2 tbsp pine nuts, roasted

2 tbsp fresh parsley, chopped

Instructions:

Preheat the oven to 400 degrees F. Place squash in the microwave for 3-4 minutes to soften. Using a sharp knife cut the squash in half lengthwise. Scoop out the seeds and discard.

Place the halves, with the cut side up, on a rimmed baking sheet. Drizzle with olive oil and sprinkle with low sodium salt and pepper.

Roast in the oven for 45-50 minutes, until you can poke the squash easily with a fork. Let cool until you can handle it safely.

Meanwhile, prepare the kale by removing the center stems and either tearing or cutting up the leaves. Heat the olive oil in a large skillet over medium heat.

Add the onion and garlic and sauté for 4-5 minutes. Add the turkey. Cook for 10-12 minutes, stirring regularly, until the turkey is browned and cooked through.

Add the kale and stir. Cook for a few minutes more to wilt the kale. Remove from heat and set aside.

Once cooled, scrape the insides of the spaghetti squash with a fork to shred the squash into strands. Transfer the strands into the skillet with the turkey and toss to combine.

Season to taste with low sodium salt and pepper. Divide the mixture among the squash shells, and then top with pine nuts and parsley to serve.

38. Delicious Turkey Veggie Lasagna

Ingredients:

For the meat sauce:

1 large yellow onion, coarsely chopped

2 cloves garlic, coarsely chopped

2 tbsp extra virgin olive oil

1 1/2 lbs. ground turkey

1/2 cup tomato paste

1/2 cup tomato sauce

1 cup red wine

1 bay leaf

3 sprigs thyme

low sodium salt and freshly ground pepper, to taste

For the lasagna:

1 eggplant, sliced lengthwise thinly

1 tsp low sodium salt

1 tbsp extra virgin olive oil

2 yellow squash, sliced thinly

1/2 cup torn fresh basil leaves

8 oz. white mushrooms, sliced

2 cups fresh spinach

2 large zucchini, sliced lengthwise into ribbons

For the topping:

1/2 head cauliflower

1 tbsp olive oil

1/2 tsp garlic powder

1/2 tsp low sodium salt

Freshly ground pepper, to taste

Instructions:

To make the meat sauce, place the onion and garlic in a food processor and pulse to finely chop.

Heat the olive oil in a heavy-bottomed saucepan over medium heat. Add the onion and garlic and season with low sodium salt and pepper. Cook for 12-15 minutes until beginning to brown, stirring frequently.

Add the turkey to the pot and season with low sodium salt and pepper.

Cook for 15 minutes until browned. Stir in the tomato paste and cook for 2-3 minutes. Add the red wine to the pan and cook for 5 more minutes.

Add the tomato sauce, bay leaf, and thyme to the pan. Bring to a simmer, and then add 1/2 cup water.

Cook at a low simmer for 1 hour, stirring occasionally and adding more water if necessary. Adjust seasonings to taste. Discard the bay leaf and thyme.

Preheat the oven to 350 degrees F. Sprinkle the eggplant with low sodium salt and set aside for 15 minutes to drain. Rinse and pat dry.

Heat one tablespoon of olive oil in a skillet over medium heat. Cook the eggplant for 2-3 minutes per side until golden.

Layer the lasagna in a baking dish. Start by layering the yellow squash as the base. Add one third of the meat sauce on top of that, then lay the eggplant slices, fresh basil, and mushrooms.

Next add the rest of the meat sauce, then the spinach, zucchini, and finally drizzle with olive oil and sprinkle with low sodium salt and pepper. Bake for 40-45 minutes.

While the lasagna is baking, place the cauliflower in a blender and process until it reaches a rice-like consistency.

Add to a skillet and sauté with the olive oil, garlic powder, low sodium salt, and pepper over medium heat.

Cook for 6-8 minutes until soft, adding a tablespoon of water if necessary. After the lasagna has cooked for 20 minutes, sprinkle with the cauliflower and return to the oven for the remaining cooking time. Serve hot.

39. Ostrich Steak or Venison with Divine Mustard Sauce and Roasted Tomatoes

Ingredients:

For the tomatoes:

2 pints cherry tomatoes, halved

2 tbsp extra virgin olive oil

Stevia to taste

low sodium salt and freshly ground pepper

For the cauliflower rice:

1/2 head of cauliflower, chopped coarsely

1/2 small onion, finely diced

1 tbsp coconut oil

1 tbsp fresh parsley, chopped

low sodium salt and freshly ground pepper, to taste

For the meat:

4 Ostrich or venison steaks

Extra virgin olive oil

low sodium salt and freshly ground pepper

Coconut oil, for the pan

For the sauce:

1/4 cup red onion, finely diced

1/4 cup apple cider vinegar

1 cup low sodium chicken stock

1 tbsp whole grain mustard

low sodium salt and freshly ground pepper, to taste

Instructions:

Preheat the oven to 400 degrees F. Place the tomatoes on a baking sheet and drizzle with olive oil and honey. Sprinkle with low sodium salt and pepper and toss to coat evenly. Bake for 15-20 minutes until soft.

While the tomatoes are roasting, prepare the cauliflower rice. Place the cauliflower into a food processor and pulse until reduced to the size of rice grains.

Melt the coconut oil in a nonstick skillet over medium heat. Add the onion and cook for 5-6 minutes until translucent. Stir in the cauliflower, season with low sodium salt and pepper, and cover. Cook for 7-10 minutes until the cauliflower has softened, and then toss with parsley.

To make the lamb, preheat the oven to 325 degrees F. Pat the ostrich or venison dry and rub with olive oil. Generously season both sides with low sodium salt and pepper.

Heat one tablespoon of coconut oil in a cast iron skillet. When the pan is hot, add to the pan and sear for 2-3 minutes on all sides until golden brown.

Place the skillet in the oven and bake for 5-8 minutes until the ostrich or venison reaches desired doneness. Let rest for 10 minutes before serving.

While the meat is resting, add the red onion to the skillet with the pan drippings from the lamb. Sauté for 3-4 minutes, then add the white wine vinegar.

Turn the heat to high and cook until the vinegar has mostly evaporated. Add the stock and bring to a boil, cooking until the sauce reduces by half.

Stir in the mustard, and season to taste with low sodium salt and pepper. Pour over ostrich or venison to serve.

40. Tantalizing Turkey Pepper Stir-fry

Ingredients:

2 bell peppers, sliced

1 cup broccoli florets

2 cooked and shredded turkey breasts

1/4 teaspoon chili powder

low sodium salt and pepper to taste

1 tablespoon coconut oil for frying

Instructions:

Add 1 tablespoon coconut oil into a frying pan on a medium heat.

Place the sliced bell peppers into the frying pan.

After the bell peppers soften, add in the cooked turkey meat.

Add in the chili powder, low sodium salt and pepper.

Mix well and stir-fry for a few more minutes.

41. Cheeky Chicken Stir Fry

Ingredients:

1 pound boneless, skinless chicken breast

2 tablespoons coconut oil

1 medium onion, finely chopped (about 1 cup)

2 heads broccoli, sliced into 3-inch spears (about 4 cups)

2 medium carrots, sliced (about 1 cup)

2 heads baby bok choy, sliced crosswise into 1-inch strips (about 1½ cups)

4 ounces shiitake mushrooms, stemmed and thinly sliced (about 1 cup)

1 small zucchini, sliced (about 1 cup)

½ teaspoon low sodium salt

Garlic powder to taste

1½ cups water

Instructions:

Rinse the chicken and pat dry. Cut into 1-inch cubes and transfer to a plate.

Heat the coconut oil in a large skillet over medium heat

Saute the onion for 8 to 10 minutes, until soft and translucent

Add the broccoli, carrots, and chicken and saute for 10 minutes until almost tender

Add the bok choy, mushrooms, zucchini, and low sodium salt and saute for 5 minutes

Add 1 cup of the water, cover the skillet, and cook for about 10 minutes, until the vegetables are wilted

In a small bowl, dissolve the arrowroot powder in the remaining ½ cup of water, stirring until thoroughly combined

Season at the end with garlic powder, salt and if you like some chilli powder

42. Perfect Turkey Stir-Fry
Ingredients:

2 tbsp. of coconut oil

2 cloves of garlic (thinly sliced)

1 inch ginger (finely grated)

2-3 green (spring) onions (sliced into long slivers)

1 carrot (coarsely grated)

1 green pepper (sliced into thin, long pieces)

1 turkey breast (cut into bite-sized pieces)

1/4 cup water

2 tbsp. homemade veggie broth

A few drops of toasted sesame oil

Instructions:

Put a pot with a bit of low sodium salt to boil and make sure your rice noodles are handy. Later, when the water has boiled, pop the noodles in and give it a stir.

Heat 2 tbsp. coconut oil in a wok or large pan.

Add the sliced garlic and grated ginger to the wok and stir-fry for 30 seconds.

Add the green onion and stir-fry 1 more minute.

Add the carrot and stir-fry about a minute. You want it just barely cooked, not limp and soggy. Remove the vegetable mixture to a bowl and set aside.

Add another 2/3 tbsp. of coconut oil to the wok.

When the oil is very hot, add the green pepper and stir-fry for 1 minute.

Heat a ½ tbsp. of coconut oil, then add the pieces of turkey breast and stir-fry. I found that the turkey got some color from the previous ingredients that were in the wok. If this doesn't happen, add a tiny amount of soy sauce.

Stir-fry until just done and no more. To check, I like to cut open the biggest piece to make sure it isn't pink in the middle.

Add the sesame oil.

43. Creamy Curry Stir Fry
Ingredients:

2 cooked chicken breasts (small) or 3-4 thighs/legs

3 carrots, chopped

3 sticks celery, chopped

1-2 heads broccoli, chopped

1/2 medium onion, chopped

2 cloves garlic 1/2c coconut milk

1/2c almond or coconut milk

2 tbsp turmeric

2 tbsp curry powder

2 tbsp coconut oil

Instructions:

Put coconut oil in pan and add chopped onion. Cook until onion softens up, add garlic and cook for an additional few minutes.

Next up, add in the carrots, celery, and broccoli. Cook until they have softened a bit (but are not fully cooked).

Shred the cooked chicken up into small pieces for the stir fry and add the coconut milk, other milk, and curry spices.

Stir everything thoroughly, simmer for 5-10 minutes or until everything is cooked to your liking, and serve hot.

Add cauliflower rice (grated cauliflower boiled for 3 minutes)

44. Sexy Turkey Scramble
Ingredients:

1 pound ground turkey

2 medium yellow onions

2 bell peppers (any color)

2 medium squash or zucchini

1 large hand-full of fresh spinach (2-3 ounces)

Spices to taste: I used about 1 tablespoon each of: cumin, chili powder, garlic powder, low sodium salt, and fresh cilantro

Instructions:

Brown the turkey until well cooked in a large skillet or wok over medium high heat.

Remove and add thinly sliced onions, peppers, squash/zucchini to the pan and saute, stirring constantly, until starting to soften.

Return turkey to pan and add fresh spinach.

Spice to taste and continue to cook until spinach is wilted.

Remove and serve with any desired toppings.

45. Turkey Thai Basil
Ingredients:

2 lbs. leftover cooked turkey, cubed or shredded (chicken or shrimp would work too)

3 Tbsp fish sauce

3 Tbsp coconut aminos (or wheat free tamari)

1 Tbsp water

Stevia to taste

1 tsp low sodium salt

1/2 tsp ground white pepper

2 Tbsp coconut oil

4 baby bok choy, leaves pulled apart, hearts halved

1 red bell pepper, sliced

1 yellow bell pepper, sliced

1 large onion, sliced

3 cloves garlic, minced

1 1/2 C lightly pack Thai basil leaves

Instructions:

In a medium bowl, combine turkey with fish sauce, water, low sodium salt and pepper; stir until turkey is thoroughly coated and set aside

Melt coconut oil in large wok or frying pan over medium-high heat

Add bok choy, peppers, onion and garlic and saute until softened, about 8 minutes, stirring frequently

Add contents of set-aside bowl (with the meat) to pan and stir for about 3 minutes until turkey is fully incorporated and heated through

Remove from heat and add Thai basil, stirring until basil wilts

46. Chicken Fennel Stir-Fry
Ingredients:

3 chicken breasts or the meat from 1 whole roasted chicken

2 tablespoons coconut oil

1 onion

1 bulb of fennel

1 teaspoon each of low sodium salt, pepper, garlic powder and basil

Instructions:

Stovetop:

Cut the chicken into bite sized pieces. If chicken is raw, heat butter/coconut oil in large skillet or wok until melted.

Add chicken and cook on medium/high heat until chicken is cooked through. (If chicken is pre-cooked, cook the vegetables first then add chicken)

While cooking, cut the onion into bite sized pieces (1/2 inch) and thinly slice the fennel bulb into thin slivers.

Add all to skillet or wok, add spices and continue sautéing until all are cooked through and fragrant.

This will take approximately 10-12 minutes.

47. Moroccan Madness

Ingredients:

1 chicken breast, chopped into pieces

1/2 tbsp olive oil

1/2 onion, chopped

1 bell pepper, chopped

1 cup diced courgette

2 cloves garlic, minced

1 tsp ginger, minced

1 tsp cumin

1 tsp turmeric

1/2 tsp paprika

1/2 tbsp oregano

1/2 can diced tomatoes

1/2 cup low sodium chicken stock

low sodium salt and pepper

Instructions:

In a pan cook the chicken in the olive oil

Once it's finished cooking, remove from pan and set aside

Add to the pan the bell pepper, onion, courgette, garlic, ginger and all spices, sauté until bell pepper and onion become soft

Add back in the chicken along with the diced tomatoes and chicken stock, let simmer for 1o minutes

48. Golden Glazed Drumsticks

Ingredients:

8 medium chicken drumsticks, skin removed

olive oil spray 1 cup water

1/3 cup rice vinegar

1/3 cup low sodium gluten free soy sauce

4 drops stevia

3 cloves garlic, crushed

1 tsp ginger, grated

2 tbsp chives or scallions, chopped

1 tsp sesame seeds

Instructions:

In a heavy large saucepan, brown chicken on high for 3-4 minutes with a little spray oil. Add water, vinegar, soy sauce, stevia, garlic, ginger and cook on high until liquid comes to a boil.

Reduce heat to low and simmer, covered for about 20 minutes.

Remove cover and bring heat to high, allowing sauce to reduce down, about 8-10 minutes, until it becomes thick, turning chicken occasionally. (Keep an eye on glaze, you don't want it to burn when it start becoming thick) Transfer chicken to a platter and pour sauce on top.

Top with chives and sesame seeds and serve.

49. Spicy Grilled Turkey Recipe

Ingredients:

6 thin turkey fillets (3 oz each)

For the Marinade:

2 tbsp lemon juice

2 tbsp toasted sesame seeds

2 cloves garlic, minced

2 tsp fresh ginger, peeled and minced

2 green onions, minced

1/4 cup low sodium soy sauce (for gluten free, use tamari)

Stevia to taste

2 tsp sesame oil

Instructions:

Combine all marinade ingredients in a small bowl. Pour the mixture over the turkey, turn the pieces to coat evenly, cover and place in refrigerator a minimum of three hours, but preferably overnight.

Preheat grill to high. Grill one side first until well browned charred, about 5 minutes, turn and cook on the second side about 3 more minutes. Transfer to a serving platter.

50. Piquant Peanut Chicken
Ingredients:

3/4 cup green onion, chopped

1 1/4 cups shredded carrots

1 1/4 cups cup shredded broccoli slaw

1 cup bean bean sprouts

2 tbsp chopped salt free peanuts

1 lime, sliced

cilantro for garnish (optional)

For the Peanut Sauce:

14.5 oz fat free chicken broth

5 tbsp peanut butter

Stevia to taste

2 tbsp soy sauce (use Tamari for gluten free)

1 tbsp freshly grated ginger

2 cloves garlic, minced

For the chicken:

16 oz chicken breast, cut into thin strips

Low sodium salt and pepper (to taste)

1 tspn chilli flakes

juice of 1/2 lime

5 cloves garlic, crushed

1 tbsp fresh ginger, grated

1 tbsp soy sauce (use Tamari for gluten free)

1/2 tbsp sesame oil

Instructions:

For the peanut sauce: Combine 1 cup chicken broth, peanut butter, stevia, 2 tbsp soy sauce, ginger, and 3 cloves crushed garlic in a small saucepan and simmer over medium-low heat stirring occasionally until sauce becomes smooth and well blended, about 5-10 minutes. Set aside.

Season chicken with low sodium salt and pepper, chilli, lime, garlic, ginger and soy sauce.

Heat a large skillet or wok until hot. Add oil and sauté chicken on high heat until cooked through, about 2-3 minutes; remove from heat and set aside.

Add 2 cloves crushed garlic, scallions, carrots, broccoli slaw and/or bean sprouts and low sodium salt, sauté until tender crisp, about 1-2 minutes.

Divide chicken between 6 bowls, top with sauteed vegetables, bean sprouts, chopped peanuts (or you can toss everything together to hide the vegetables so your family members don't push them aside!) and garnish with cilantro and lime wedges.

51. Cheeky Chicken Salad

Ingredients:

olive oil spray

2 tsp olive oil

16 oz (2 large) skinless boneless chicken breasts, cut into 24 1-inch chunks

Low sodium salt and pepper to taste

4 cups shredded romaine

1 cup shredded red cabbage

For the Skinny Cheeky Sauce:

2 1/2 tbsp paleo mayonnaise

2 tbsp scallions, chopped fine plus more for topping

1 1/2 tsp chilli flakes

Instructions:

Preheat oven to 425°F. Spray a baking sheet with olive oil spray.

Season chicken with low sodium salt and pepper, olive oil and mix well so the olive oil evenly coats all of the chicken.

Meanwhile combine the sauce in a medium bowl. When the chicken is ready, drizzle it over the top and enjoy!!

52. Melting Mustard Chicken

Ingredients:

8 small chicken thighs, skin removed

3 tsp mustard powder

1 tbsp paleo mayonnaise

1 clove garlic, crushed

1 lime, squeezed, and lime zest

3/4 tsp pepper

Low sodium salt

dried parsley

Instructions:

Preheat oven to 400°. Rinse the chicken and remove the skin and all fat. Pat dry ...place in a large bowl and season generously with low sodium salt. In a small bowl combine mustard, mayonnaise, lime juice, lime zest, garlic and pepper. Mix well. Pour over chicken, tossing well to coat.

Spray a large baking pan with a little Pam to prevent sticking since all the fat and skin was removed from chicken. Place chicken to fit in a single layer.

Top the chicken with dried parsley. Bake until cooked through, about 30-35 minutes.

Finish the chicken under the broiler until it is golden brown. Serve chicken with the pan juices drizzled over the top.

53. Tantalizing Turkey with Roasted Vegetables
Ingredients:

10 (20 oz) Turkey Breasts

20 medium asparagus, ends trimmed, cut in half

3 red bell peppers

1 cup carrots, sliced in half long way

2 red onions, chopped in large chunks

10 oz sliced mushrooms

1/2 cup plus 2 tbsp rice vinegar

1/4 cup extra virgin olive oil

1 tsp stevia

Low sodium salt and pepper

3 tbsp fresh rosemary

2 cloves garlic, smashed and sliced

2 tbsp oregano or thyme

4 leaves fresh sage, chopped

Instructions:

Preheat oven to 425°. Wash and dry the chicken well with a paper towel. Combine all the ingredients together and using your hands and arrange in a very large roasting pan.

The vegetables should not touch the turkey or it will steam instead of roast.

All ingredients should be spread out in a single layer. If necessary use two baking sheets or disposable tins to achieve this. Bake for 35 - 40 minutes.

54. Grilled Ostrich Steak
Ingredients:

6 medium ostrich steaks

1 tbsp vinegar

garlic powder

black pepper ground to taste

oregano

2 tablespoons olive oil

Instructions:

Season ostrich with vinegar and olive oil.

Add garlic powder, oregano and mix well....marinate at least 20 minutes.

Broil or grill on low until ostrich is cooked through, careful not to burn. Enjoy with green salad.

55. Lemony Chicken and Asparagus

Ingredients:

1 1/2 pounds skinless chicken breast, cut into 1-inch cubes

Low sodium salt, to taste

1/2 cup reduced-sodium chicken broth

2 tablespoons reduced-sodium soy sauce (or Tamari for GF)

2 tablespoons water

1 tbsp olive oil, divided

1 bunch asparagus, ends trimmed, cut into 2-inch pieces

6 cloves garlic, chopped

1 tbsp fresh ginger

3 tablespoons fresh lemon juice

fresh black pepper, to taste

Instructions:

Lightly season the chicken with low sodium salt. In a small bowl, combine chicken broth and soy sauce. In a second small bowl combine the cornstarch and water and mix well to combine.

Heat a large non-stick wok over medium-high heat, when hot add 1 teaspoon of the oil, then add the asparagus and cook until tender-crisp, about 3 to 4 minutes. Add the garlic and ginger and cook until golden, about 1 minute. Set aside.

Increase the heat to high, then add 1 teaspoon of oil and half of the chicken and cook until browned and cooked through, about 4 minutes on each side. Remove and set aside and repeat with the remaining oil and chicken. Set aside.

Add the soy sauce mixture; bring to a boil and cook about 1-1/2 minutes. Add lemon juice and stir well, when it simmers return the chicken and asparagus to the wok and mix well, remove from heat and serve.

56. Delish Chicken Soup

Ingredients:

5 cups reduced sodium chicken broth

2 cups shredded chicken breast

1 tomato, diced

2 cloves garlic, minced

1-1/2 cups scallions, chopped fine

1/3 cup cilantro, chopped fine

4 lime wedges

2 tsp olive oil

Low sodium salt and fresh pepper to taste

pinch cumin

pinch chile powder (optional)

Instructions:

In a large pot, heat oil over medium heat. Add 1 cup of scallions and garlic. Sauté about 2 minutes then add tomatoes and sauté another minute, until soft.

Add chicken stock, cumin and chile powder and bring to a boil. Simmer, covered on low for about 15-20 minutes.

Ladle 1 cup chicken broth over the chicken and serve with a lime wedge.

57. Chicken Paprika Surprise

Ingredients:

1 lb iced paprika – use all 4 colours

12 oz (3) boneless skinless chicken thighs, all fat trimmed

8 cups water

1 tbsp low salt chicken Bouillon

1 small onion

2 scallions

1/4 cup chopped cilantro

3 cloves garlic

1 medium ripe tomato

1 tsp garlic powder

1 tsp cumin

1/4 tsp oregano

1/4 tsp ground Spanish paprika

Low sodium salt, to taste

Instructions:

In a large pot combine paprikas, chicken, water and chicken bouillon. Bring to a boil, covered over medium-low heat until chicken is cooked, about 20 minutes. Remove the chicken and shred, return to the pot.

Meanwhile, in a chopper or by hand, mince the onions, scallions, cilantro, garlic, and tomato. Add to the lentils with garlic powder, cumin, oregano and cook, covered until the lentils are soft, about 25 more minutes, adding more water as needed if too thick. Adjust low sodium salt to taste as needed.

58. Chicken Healing Soup
Ingredients:

1 teaspoon olive oil

1 cup chopped carrots

1 cup chopped onions

1/2 cup chopped celery

2 cloves garlic, chopped

1-1/2 lbs skinless bone-in chicken breast (makes 14 oz cooked)

7 cups reduced sodium chicken broth

1/4 cup chopped parsley

2 bay leaves

fresh ground black pepper, to taste

Instructions:

Heat a large heavy pot on medium heat. Add the oil, carrots, onion, celery and garlic to the pot and stir.

Add chicken, broth, parsley, and bay leaves and bring to a boil. When boiling, reduce heat to low and cover.

Simmer covered over low heat until the chicken and vegetables are tender, about 30 minutes.

Remove the chicken, shred or cut the meat, discard the bones and return the chicken to the pot along with the barley, adjust the low sodium salt if needed and add fresh ground pepper.

Simmer for 20 minutes…. Discard the bay leaves and serve.

59. Chicken a la King
Ingredients:

6 chicken thighs, skin and fat removed

olive oil spray

1 red bell pepper, chopped

1 cup chopped mushrooms

1/2 onion, chopped

2 garlic cloves, finely chopped

1 (28-ounce) can crushed tomatoes

1/4 cup fat free chicken broth, more if needed

1 tsp dried oregano leaves

1/4 cup fresh chopped basil leaves

Low sodium salt and freshly ground black pepper

Instructions:

Season chicken with low sodium salt and pepper. In a large heavy saute pan, heat the pan over a medium-high flame and spray with cooking oil.

Add the chicken pieces to the pan and saute just until brown, about 3-4 minutes per side.

Add the peppers, onion and garlic to the pan and saute over medium heat until the onion is tender, about 3-4 minutes, then add mushrooms and cook another 2-3 minutes. Season with low sodium salt and pepper. Add the tomatoes, broth, and oregano.

Cover the pan and bring the sauce to a simmer. Continue simmering over low heat until the chicken is just cooked through, about 25 minutes.

Add the chopped basil 5 minutes before sauce is done.

Option – serve with cauliflower rice!;

60. Chicken Coconut Divine

Ingredients:

1 tbsp olive oil

1/2 tsp roasted cumin

1-1/2 tsp garam masala

2 tsp curry powder

1/2 onion, minced

5 cloves garlic, minced

1 large tomato, chopped

2 tbsp fresh cilantro, chopped

1/2 cup light coconut milk

3/4 cup water

6 skinless chicken thighs

Low sodium salt to taste

Instructions:

Add oil to a large pan, on medium heat. When oil is hot add onion and garlic and sauté. Add cumin, masala and curry powder and mix well.

Place chicken in the pan and season with low sodium salt. Mix together with all spices and brown on both side for a few minutes.

Add tomatoes, cilantro, water, coconut milk and adjust low sodium salt to taste. Mix all ingredients and cover pan, simmer on low until chicken is cooked through, about 20 minutes.

Option ...Serve with Cauliflower rice

61. Skinny Turkey Lettuce Fajitas

Ingredients:

16 oz turkey breasts

1 red bell pepper, cut into strips

1 green pepper, cut into strips

1 medium onion, cut into strips

3 tbsp lime juice

1 tsp ground cumin

1 tsp garlic powder

Pinch chile powder, to taste

low sodium salt and pepper to taste

2 tsp olive oil

8 Large Lettuce cups (iceberg)

Instructions:

Marinate the turkey with lime juice, and season with chile powder, low sodium salt, pepper, garlic powder and cumin.

Season vegetables with low sodium salt and pepper and toss with olive oil. To grill the onions and peppers outside on the grill, use a cast iron skillet and grill covered over medium heat until tender, about 15 minutes.

Or, to cook them indoors, you can use a large skillet on the stove over medium heat for 16 to 18 minutes, covered until the onions and peppers are soft.

Heat an outdoor grill or indoor grill pan over medium heat; grill turkey until cooked through, about 8 minutes on each side. Transfer to a cutting board when done and cut into strips. Once cooked, combine with the peppers and onions. Serve immediately inside lettuce cups.

62. Chicken Jerez

Ingredients:

4 large (32 oz) chicken breast halves, thinly sliced in 3 (12 cutlets total)

1 large lemon, juice of (about 3 tbsp) or more, to taste

1/2 lemon sliced thin

1/3 cup Jerez Sherry

15 oz low sodium chicken broth

cooking spray

low sodium salt and fresh pepper, to taste

3 tbsp fresh chopped parsley

1 tbsp olive oil

Instructions:

Season the chicken with low sodium salt and pepper. Heat a very large non stick pan over medium heat. When hot spray with cooking spray to lightly coat the bottom of the pan.

Saute chicken 2-3 minutes on each side. When cooked, transfer onto a plate. Spray the pan again and repeat until all chicken has been cooked.

Once all chicken is cooked, place the chicken broth in the bowl and to the pan along with the juice of the lemon, sherry, lemon slices, parsley and butter and simmer over medium heat for about 2 minutes so it reduces slightly. Turn off heat. Return chicken to the pan to combine with the sauce. Serve immediately with steamed vegetables of choice.

63. Leeky Chicken

Ingredients:

1 or 2 leeks (3/4 cup) white part and light green only

16 oz (6) skinless chicken breast cutlets, sliced thin

2 tsp olive oil, divided

1 clove garlic, minced

2 oz ready-to-eat sun dried tomatoes (not in oil), sliced

1/4 cup white wine

1/2 cup fat free low sodium chicken broth

Low sodium salt and fresh pepper to taste

2 tbsp chopped fresh parsley

Instructions:

Cut off green tops of leek and remove outer tough leaves. Cut off root and cut leeks in half lengthwise. Fan out the leeks and rinse well under running water, leaving them intact. Slice leeks into 1/4-inch slices. Set aside.

Preheat oven to 200°. Season chicken with low sodium salt and pepper. Heat a large skillet on medium heat; when hot add 1tsp olive oil. Add chicken to the skillet and cook on medium heat for about 3 - 4 minutes on each side, or until chicken is no longer pink. Set aside in a warm oven.

Add additional oil to the skillet, then garlic and cook a few seconds; add leeks, low sodium salt and pepper. Sauté stirring occasionally until golden, about 5 minutes.

Add sun dried tomatoes, wine, chicken broth, parsley; stir the pan with a wooden spoon, breaking up any brown bits from the bottom of the pan. Cook 2 more minutes or until the liquid reduces almost by half. Top the chicken with the sun dried tomato/leeks mixture and serve with a green salad

64. Zesty Chicken Lemon

Ingredients:

2 (16 oz total) skinless chicken breasts, all fat trimmed

freshly ground black pepper

2 large egg whites

olive oil 2 tablespoons and spray (about 1 tbsp worth)

juice of 2 lemons, lemon halves reserved

1/4 cup dry white wine

1/2 cup reduced sodium chicken broth

1 tbsp capers

Sliced lemon, for serving

Chopped fresh parsley leaves, for serving

Instructions:

Cut chicken into 4 cutlets, then place cutlets between 2 sheets of parchment paper or plastic wrap and pound out to 1/4-inch thick. Sprinkle both sides with low sodium salt and pepper.

Heat a large saute pan over medium to medium-low heat. Spray a generous amount of olive oil spray on one side of the chicken, and lay it in the pan, oil side down. Spray the top of the chicken generously to coat and cook for 2-3 minutes on each side, until cooked through. Set aside until you make the sauce.

For the sauce, clean the saute pan. Over medium heat, add olive oil, add the lemon juice, wine, chicken broth and the reserved lemon halves, low sodium salt, and pepper. Boil over high heat until reduced in half, about 2 minutes. Discard the lemon halves, add the capers and serve one chicken cutlet on each plate. Spoon on the sauce and serve with a slice of lemon and a sprinkling of fresh parsley.

Serve with any steamed vegetables!

65. Sweety Chicky Soup
Ingredients:

2 (26 oz) chicken breasts, on the bone, skin removed

1 teaspoon seasoning low sodium salt

1/2 tsp olive oil

1 large onion, chopped

2 celery stalks, chopped

3 garlic cloves, chopped

1/2 tsp dried oregano

1/2 tsp dried thyme

1/2 tsp ground cumin

6 cups reduced sodium chicken broth

1 large sweet potato, peeled and diced 1-inch cubes

3 cups kale, roughly chopped

1 fresh jalapeno, sliced in half lengthwise

1/4 cup fresh cilantro

Instructions:

Season the chicken with the salt and set aside while you prep all your vegetables.

Heat a large nonstick pot over medium-low heat, add the oil and the onions and celery and cook until soft and golden, about 8 to 10 minutes, then add the garlic and dry spices and cook 2 to 3 minutes.

Add the chicken broth, chicken, jalapeno and cilantro. Cover and cook 20 minutes, then add the sweet potato and kale and cook until the sweet potatoes are tender and the chicken is cooked, about 25 to 30 minutes.

Remove the chicken, shred or cut up and discard the bones. Return to the pot, discard the jalapeno and serve the soup into 6 bowls.

66. Chicken Zoodle Delish
Ingredients:

For the sauce:

1/2 cup reduced sodium chicken broth

1 tbsp reduced sodium soy sauce gluten free

1/2 tbsp rice wine

For the zoodles:

2 medium zucchini, ends trimmed

8 oz skinless, boneless chicken breast, cut into thin short strips

Low sodium salt, to taste

2 tsp olive oil, divided

3/4 cup sliced bok choy

1/2 cup sliced mushrooms such as shiitake

1/2 cup shredded carrots

3 scallions, sliced into 1-inch pieces on the diagonal

1/2 tbsp grated fresh ginger

2 garlic cloves, chopped

1 tablespoon almond flour

Instructions:

For the sauce – in a medium bowl, combine the chicken broth, soy sauce and 2 tablespoons of water. Use 1 tablespoon almond flour to thicken

Using a spiralizer fitted with a shredder blade, or a mandolin fitted with a julienne blade, cut the zucchini into long spaghetti-like strips. If using a spiralizer, use kitchen scissors to cut the strands into pieces that are about 8 inches long so they're easier to eat.

Season chicken with low sodium salt. Heat a large nonstick wok over high heat. When very hot, add 1 tsp of the oil and the chicken. Cook until browned on both sides and opaque throughout, 2 to 3 minutes. Set aside.

Add the remaining oil, bokchoy, mushroom, carrots, scallions, ginger and garlic. Cook until crisp tender, 2 to 3 minutes. Set aside with the chicken.

Pour the sauce mixture into the wok and cook, stirring, until thickened and bubbling, 1 to 1-1/2 minutes.

Add the zucchini noodles to the sauce, mixing so the zucchini is covered in sauce, and cook until the zucchini is tender, 2 minutes.

Add the chicken and vegetables to combine, then divide between two serving bowls.

67. Coconut Turkey Salad

Ingredients:

6 (about 12 oz) turkey breasts

6 tbsp shredded coconut

Pinch low sodium salt

olive oil spray

6 cups mixed baby greens

3/4 cup shredded carrots

1 large tomato, sliced

1 small cucumber, sliced

2 beaten egg whites organic

For the Vinaigrette:

1 tbsp oil

Stevia to taste

1 tbsp white vinegar

2 tsp mustard powder

Instructions:

Whisk all vinaigrette ingredients; set aside.

Preheat oven to 375°.

Combine coconut flakes and low sodium salt in a bowl. Put egg whites or egg beaters in another bowl.

Lightly season chicken with low sodium salt. Dip the chicken in the egg, then in the coconut flake mixture. Place chicken on a cookie sheet lined with parchment for easy cleanup. Lightly spray with olive oil spray and bake for 30 minutes turning halfway, or until chicken is cooked through.

Place 2 cups baby greens on each plate. Divide carrots, cucumber, tomato evenly between each plate. When chicken is ready slice on the diagonal and place on top of greens. Heat dressing and divide equally between each salad; a little over 1 tbsp each.

68. Creamy Chicken Mushroom Soup Bonanza

Ingredients:

4 cups water

1 celery stalk, cut in half

5 oz shiitake mushrooms, sliced

4 tsp Chicken Bouillon (low salt)

7 oz skinless chicken breast

1 tbsp fresh parsley, chopped

1 tablespoon almond flour

Instructions:

Place cold water and flour in a blender and blend until smooth; pour into a medium pot and set heat to medium.

Add celery, mushrooms, chicken bouillon and bring to a boil. Add chicken, cover and simmer on low 15 minutes, or until chicken is cooked through.

Remove chicken and set aside; continue to cook the remaining soup an additional 5 minutes, until vegetables are soft.

Place celery and 1 cup of soup into the blender; blend until smooth, then return to the pot and simmer a few minutes. Shred or cut the chicken into small pieces and add back to the soup, garnish with fresh parsley.

69. Feisty Filipino Chicken

Ingredients:

8 chicken legs on the bone (skin removed)

1/3 cup low sodium soy sauce

1/3 cup apple cider vinegar

1 small head of garlic, crushed

6 ground peppercorns

4 bay leaves

1 jalapeño, chopped (optional)

Instructions:

Marinate chicken in vinegar, soy sauce, garlic, jalapeño and pepper, for at least an hour (overnight is ideal).

Add chicken, 1/2 cup water, bay leaves and marinade into a deep nonstick skillet and cook on medium-low heat. Cover and cook until the meat is tender, about 45 minutes.

Remove the cover and cook an additional 15 minutes, until the sauce reduces. Discard bay leaves and serve over cauliflower rice.

70. Chinese Chicken Legs

Ingredients:

3 lbs (6) chicken legs (thighs and legs attached), fat trimmed

For the marinade:

6 cloves of garlic

1 large shallot

1 tbsp grated fresh ginger

Stevia to taste

1/4 cup reduced sodium soy sauce (tamari for gluten free)

1/2 tsp Chinese five-spice powder

freshly ground black pepper

Instructions:

In a blender combine the marinade ingredients; blend until smooth.

Place the chicken in a large, resealable zip-top bag or container and pour in the marinade. Toss the chicken inside the bag to cover evenly with the marinade and refrigerate for 6-8 hours or as long as overnight.

Preheat oven to 400°F. Place the chicken on a rack in a foil lined roasting pan. Create a loose tent over the chicken with foil.

Roast the chicken in the center of the oven 30 minutes; remove foil and continue to cook, basting occasionally until the internal temperature is 165°-170°F, about 45 minutes longer (Insert thermometer between the leg and the thigh).

Serve with green salad

71. Jolly Jamaican Chicken

Ingredients:

6 bone-in chicken legs with thighs attached, skin removed (6 thighs, 6 drumsticks)

1 lime or 1/4 cup lime juice

1 large tomato, chopped

4 medium scallions, chopped

1 large onion, chopped

2 garlic cloves, chopped

1/2 - 1 hot chilli, chopped

4 sprigs fresh thyme or 2 tsp dried thyme

2 tbsp low sodium soy sauce (for gluten free use GF Tamari)

1 tsp coconut oil 1 medium carrot, chopped finely

2 tsp almond flour

1 1/2 cups unsweetened light coconut milk

1/4 tsp low sodium salt

Instructions:

Squeeze lime over chicken and rub well. Drain off excess lime juice.

Using gloves combine tomato, scallion, onion, garlic, chilli pepper, thyme and soy sauce in a large bowl and add to the chicken. Cover and marinate at least one hour.

Heat oil in a large saucepan. Shake off the seasonings as you remove each piece of chicken from the marinade, reserving the marinade for later.

Lightly brown the chicken on medium-high heat. When browned on all sides, pour the marinade over the chicken and add the carrots. Stir and cook over medium heat for 10 minutes.

Mix flour and coconut milk and add to stew, stirring constantly. Reduce heat to low and cook an additional 20 minutes or until tender, add low sodium salt to taste.

72. Citrus Chicken
Ingredients:

For the e Sauce:

1/3 cup freshly-squeezed lemon juice

1/4 cup reduced sodium chicken broth

2 tbsp soy sauce (Tamari for gluten-free)

Stevia to taste

1 tbsp Chinese rice wine

Chilli flakes to taste

1 tbsp rice vinegar

1/4 teaspoon white pepper

For the chicken:

20 oz skinless, boneless chicken breast, cut into small cubes

Low sodium salt, to taste

1 tbsp sesame oil

4 cloves minced garlic

1-inch grated ginger

1 teaspoon grated lemon zest

2 tbsp chopped scallions

1/2 tsp sesame seeds, for garnish

Instructions:

Mix the lemon sauce ingredients and set aside.

Season the chicken lightly with low sodium salt and coat evenly with corn starch, set aside.

Heat a wok on high heat, add 1 teaspoon of sesame oil and add half of the chicken. Cook 2 to 3 minutes on each side until well browned, set aside. Add 1 teaspoon of oil and chicken and repeat cooking 2 to 3 minutes on each side. Set aside with the rest of the chicken.

Add remaining teaspoon of oil and quickly stir-fry the minced garlic and ginger until fragrant, about 1 minute. Add the orange zest then return the chicken to the pan. Quickly stir the chicken then add the sauce and cook until the sauce thickens, about 1 to 2 minutes. Divide between 4 plates and garnish with the scallion and sesame seeds.

73. Beautiful Baked Chicken
Ingredients:

6 medium bone-in skinless drumsticks

3 tsp low sodium salt

1/2 tsp garlic powder

1/2 tsp paprika

1/2 tsp fresh black pepper

1/2 tsp cayenne pepper

5 tbsp paleo mayonnaise

1 tsp mustard powder

Oil spray

2 teaspoons almond flour

Instructions:

Preheat oven to 400°. Line a baking sheet with foil and set a rack above. Spray rack with oil.

Crush cereal in a food processor or chopper. In a bowl mix almond flour with low sodium salt, paprika, garlic powder, black pepper and cayenne pepper. Place in a shallow dish or ziplock bag.

Combine mayonnaise and mustard. Using a cooking brush, brush onto chicken then coat chicken with crushed cereal mixture. Place chicken on wire rack and spray with oil. Bake 35-40 minutes.

74. South American Chicken

Ingredients:

1 whole chicken

1/4 cup white vinegar

1 lime, juice of

2 tsp cumin

2 tsp garlic powder

1 tsp dried oregano

Low sodium salt

paprika

Sauce:

2-3 jalapeños, seeded

3 tbsp fresh cilantro

2 tbsp olive oil

1 clove garlic

1 tbsp white vinegar

pinch cumin

low sodium salt and pepper

2 tbsp coconut cream

Instructions:

For Sauce: Place all ingredients in a blender and puree until smooth.

Wash chicken and remove all fat. Place in a large bowl and season generously with beer, vinegar, lime juice, low sodium salt, garlic powder, cumin and oregano. Place in a large bag and marinate overnight.

Remove chicken from bag, cut chicken in half and place both halves on a large oven safe baking dish, skin side up. Discard marinade. Sprinkle chicken with paprika and a little more garlic powder and low sodium salt and bake at 425° for about 50 minutes, basting with the pan juices half way through.

75. Rosemary Chicken
Ingredients:

1 (3 lb) chicken, washed and dried, fat removed

1/2 onion, chopped in large chunks

2 cloves garlic, smashed

1/2 lemon

2-3 sprigs rosemary

1 tbsp herbes de Provence (or dried rosemary)

Low sodium salt and fresh pepper

Instructions:

Heat oven to 425°. Season chicken inside and out with low sodium salt, pepper, and herbs de provence. Squeeze lemon juice on the outside of the chicken and stuff the remains of the lemon along with onion, garlic, rosemary sprigs inside the chicken.

Roast the chicken until the internal temperature is 165°F, about 50-60 minutes (Insert thermometer between the leg and the thigh). Let the bird rest for 10 minutes before carving.

Serve with steamed vegetables of choice

76. Sexy Sesame Turkey
Ingredients:

18 oz turkey breasts

Low sodium salt and pepper to taste

2 tsp sesame oil

2 tsp low sodium soy sauce gluten free

6 tbsp toasted sesame seeds

1/2 tsp low sodium salt

olive oil 2 teaspoons and spray

Instructions:

Preheat oven to 425°. Spray a baking sheet with non-stick oil spray.

Combine the sesame oil and soy sauce in a bowl, and the sesame seeds and low sodium salt.

Place turkey in the bowl with the oil and soy sauce, then into the sesame seed mixture to coat well. Place on the baking sheet; lightly spray the top of the chicken with oil spray and bake 8 - 10 minutes. Turn over and cook another 4 - 5 minutes longer or until cooked through.

Serve with cauliflower rice or fried celeriac

77. Pollo Al Vinagre
Ingredients:

8 lean chicken thighs, skin removed

Low sodium salt and fresh pepper

1/2 cup red wine vinegar

1 cup fat free low salt chicken broth

Stevia to taste

1 tbsp tomato paste

1 tsp butter

1 large shallot, thinly sliced (3/4 cup)

2 cloves garlic, thinly sliced

1/2 cup dry white wine

2 tbsp coconut cream

2 tbsp fresh chopped parsley

Instructions:

Season chicken with low sodium salt and pepper.

In a medium saucepan, combine vinegar, stevia, 3/4 cup chicken broth and tomato paste. Boil about 5 minutes, until it reduces down to about 3/4 cup. Remove from heat.

In a large skillet, melt butter over medium-low heat and add chicken. Cook on both sides, until brown, about 6-8 minutes. Remove chicken and set aside. Add the shallots and garlic to the skillet and cook on low until soft, about 5 minutes. Pour the sauce over the chicken, add the wine, remaining broth low sodium salt and pepper. Cover and simmer about 20 minutes until tender.

Remove the chicken, add cream and stir into the sauce (if sauce dries up, add more broth). Boil a few minutes then return chicken to skillet. Top with fresh parsley.

78. Chicken Caully Delish
Ingredients:

1 1/2 tbsp olive oil

2 large chicken breast halves, bone in, skin removed

Low sodium salt and pepper to taste

1/2 medium head of cauliflower, cut into florets (about 4 cups)

1 medium onion, sliced thinly

4 cloves of garlic, sliced thinly

1driedchilli pepper, sliced

1/3 cup dry white wine

1 cup reduced sodium chicken stock

1 sprig rosemary, needles removed and roughly chopped, plus additional for garnish

Instructions:

Pre-heat oven to 375°F. Cut chicken in half to make 4 pieces, leaving the bone on.

Heat oil in a large, oven safe sauté pan with straight sides over medium-high heat. Season the chicken with low sodium salt and pepper and brown 2-3 minutes per side. Remove chicken and set aside.

Lower heat to medium and add onion, cauliflower florets, garlic and chill ...Sauté, stirring frequently, for 2-3 minutes until vegetables start to brown.

Add the white wine, cherry peppers and additional optional liquid. Raise heat and allow to boil for about 2 minutes before adding chicken stock. Add chicken breasts back into pan, bone side down, sprinkle rosemary on top, bring to a boil and then place the pan in the oven, uncovered.

Cook for 20-25 minutes or until chicken reaches 165°F.

Remove from oven carefully, with towel or kitchen gloves, serve and enjoy!

79. Courgette Spaghetti with Delish Chicken

Ingredients:

2 skinless chicken breast halves, diced in 1 inch cubes

cooking spray

1/2 tsp each of dried oregano and dries basil

Low sodium salt and fresh pepper

2 courgettes spiralized

2 cups grape tomatoes, halved

6 cloves garlic, smashed and coarsely chopped

4 tsp extra virgin olive oil

4 tbsp chopped fresh basil

Instructions:

Bring a large pot of salted water to boil.

Season chicken generously with low sodium salt, pepper, oregano and basil. Heat a large skillet on high heat. When hot, spray with oil and add chicken. Cook about 3-4 minutes, until no longer pink. Remove chicken and set aside.

Add courgette pasta and cook according to package directions. Reserve about 1/2 cup pasta water before draining.

While pasta cooks, add olive oil to skillet on high heat. Add garlic and sauté until golden brown (do not burn). Add tomatoes, low sodium salt and pepper and reduce heat to medium-low. Sauté about 4-5 minutes. When pasta is drained, add pasta to tomatoes and toss well. If pasta seems too dry, add some of the reserved pasta water. Add fresh basil and chicken and toss well. Serve and top with dried garlic powder and the rest of the basil.

80. Chicken Pea Stir Fry

Ingredients:

For the sauce:

1 tbsp low sodium soy sauce gluten free

1 tbsp fresh lime juice

2 tbsp water

For the Stir Fry:

1 lb skinless, boneless chicken breast, sliced thin

Low sodium salt, to taste

1 tbsp sesame oil,

2 tsp fresh garlic, minced

1 tsp fresh ginger, grated

2 cups sugar snap peas

1 cup carrots, sliced diagonally

scallions for garnish

Instructions:

Combine soy sauce, lime juice, water in a small bowl, mix together and set aside.

Season chicken lightly with low sodium salt. Heat a large wok over high heat. When the wok is very hot, add half of the oil, then add the chicken. Stir fry, stirring occasionally until the chicken is cooked through and browned, about 3-4 minutes. With a slotted spoon, remove the chicken and set aside. Reduce heat to medium.

Add the remaining oil to the wok; add the garlic and ginger, stir for 20 seconds. Add the sugar snap peas and carrots, stirring over medium high heat until tender crisp, about 3-4 minutes.

Return the chicken to the wok, add the soy sauce-lime mixture, mix well and cook another 30 seconds to one minute. Serve immediately and top with fresh scallions.

81. Chicken Pineapple Delight

Ingredients:

1 lb boneless skinless chicken breast, cut into 1-inch cubes

2 tbsp cornstarch

1 tbsp oil, divided

1 tsp minced garlic

1 tsp minced ginger

2 cups cubed assorted colors bell peppers (1/2-inch cubes)

1 red chili pepper, chopped (optional or to taste)

1 cup fresh pineapple chunks

1/2 teaspoon chilli flakes...optional – this is hot!

cilantro leaves (for garnish)

Instructions:

Heat 1/2 tablespoon of the oil in large nonstick skillet on medium-high heat. Add garlic and ginger; stir fry 30 seconds. Add bell peppers, chili pepper if using and pineapple; stir fry 3 to 5 minutes or until peppers are tender-crisp. Add sauce; cook and stir until heated through. Remove from skillet.

Heat remaining oil in the skillet. Add chicken; stir fry 5 minutes or until cooked through. Return bell pepper mixture to skillet; stir fry until well blended. Garnish with cilantro.

82. Chicken Peanut Lettuce Wraps

Ingredients:

For the Peanut Sauce:

1/2 cup reduced-sodium chicken broth

3 tbsp PB2 (or 2 tbsp peanut butter)

Stevia to taste

1 tbsp soy sauce (use Tamari for gluten free)

1/2 tbsp freshly grated ginger

1 clove garlic, crushed

For the Chicken cooking spray

16 oz ground chicken

4 cloves garlic, crushed

1 tbsp fresh ginger, grated

1 tbsp soy sauce (use Tamari for gluten free)

3/4 cups shredded carrots

2/3 cup scallions, chopped

3/4 cup shredded red cabbage

2 tbsp chopped peanuts

cilantro leaves, for garnish

4 lime wedges

8 iceberg lettuces outer leaves

Instructions:

Make the peanut sauce; in a small saucepan combine chicken broth, stevia, 1 tablespoon soy sauce, 1/2 tablespoon fresh ginger, and 1 clove crushed garlic and simmer over medium-low heat stirring occasionally until sauce becomes smooth and thickens, about 6 to 8 minutes.

Meanwhile, heat a large non-stick skillet or wok over high medium until hot. When hot, spray with oil and sauté the chicken until cooked through and browned, breaking it up as it cooks; add the remaining garlic and ginger and saute 1 minute. Add the tablespoon of soy sauce, cook 1 minute.

Add the shredded carrots, and 1/2 cup of the scallions and sauté until tender crisp, about 1-2 minutes. Set aside.

Divide the chicken equally between 8 lettuce leaves, top each with shredded cabbage, remaining scallions, drizzle with peanut sauce, chopped peanuts and cilantro, for garnish and serve with lime wedges.

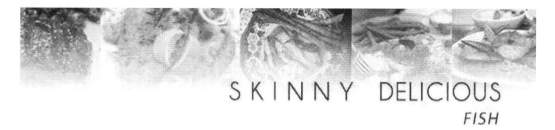

SKINNY DELICIOUS
FISH

MAIN COURSE - FISH

83. Thai Baked Fish with Squash Noodles

Ingredients:

1 medium spaghetti squash

Extra virgin olive oil, for drizzling

low sodium salt and pepper

1 tbsp coconut oil

1/2 large onion, finely chopped

1 head broccoli, de-stemmed and cut into florets

2 heads baby bok choy, sliced into 1-inch strips

4 scallions, sliced

1/4 tsp red pepper flakes

1/3 cup cashews, toasted and chopped

For the Sauce:

1 tsp lime juice

1/2-inch piece fresh ginger, peeled and minced

1 clove garlic, minced

1/2 tsp red wine vinegar

3 tbsp almond butter

3 tbsp coconut milk

For the Fish:

2 whole fish fillets...use cod or any good quality white fish

Instructions:

Preheat the oven to 400 degrees F. Place squash in the microwave for 3-4 minutes to soften. Using a sharp knife, cut the squash in half lengthwise. Scoop out the seeds and discard. Place the halves, with the cut side up, on a rimmed baking sheet. Drizzle with olive oil and sprinkle with low sodium salt and pepper. Roast in the oven for 45-50 minutes, until you can poke the squash easily with a fork. Let cool until you can handle it safely. Then scrape the insides with a fork to shred the squash into strands.

While the squash cooks, make the sauce. Combine the lime juice, ginger, garlic, and red wine vinegar in a blender or food processor until smooth. Add the almond butter and coconut milk and blend until completely combined. Adjust the levels of almond butter and coconut milk to reach desired level of creaminess.

Melt the coconut oil in a large pan over medium heat. Add the onion and cook for 5-6 minutes until translucent. Add the broccoli and sauté for 8-10 minutes, until just tender. Then stir in the bok choy and cook for 3-4 minutes until wilted. Lastly add the cooked spaghetti squash into the pan and stir to combine.

To assemble, top the spaghetti squash mixture with the scallions and cilantro. Sprinkle with roasted cashews and drizzle with Thai sauce.

Place the whole fish under the grill at 200 degrees for 25 minutes topped with a tablespoon of olive oil, fresh pressed garlic (one clove) and cayenne pepper to taste.

Finnish off the fish with a squirt of lemon juice to taste.

84. Divine Prawn Mexicana

Ingredients:

1 tbsp extra virgin olive oil

1 tsp chili powder

1 tsp low sodium salt

1 lb. medium shrimp, peeled and deveined

1 avocado, pitted and diced

Shredded lettuce, for serving

Fresh cilantro, for serving

1 lime, cut into wedges

For the tortillas:

6 egg whites

1/4 cup coconut flour

1/4 cup almond milk

1/2 tsp low sodium salt

1/2 tsp cumin

1/4 tsp chili powder

Instructions:

Combine all of the tortilla ingredients together in a small bowl and mix well. Allow the batter to sit for approximately 10 minutes to allow the flour to soak up some of the moisture, and then stir again. The consistency should be similar to crepe batter.

While the batter is resting, heat a skillet to medium-high. Mix together the olive oil, chili powder, and low sodium salt and toss with the shrimp to coat. Cook in the skillet for 1-2 minutes per side, until translucent. Set aside.

Coat the pan with coconut oil spray. Pour about 1/4 cup of batter onto the skillet, turning the pan with your wrist to help it spread out in a thin, even layer. Cook for 1-2 minutes, loosening the sides with a spatula. When the bottom has firmed up, carefully flip over and cook for another 2-3 minutes until lightly browned, then set aside on a plate. Repeat with remaining batter.

Top each tortilla with cooked shrimp, shredded lettuce, avocado, and cilantro. Serve with a lime wedge.

85. Superior Salmon with Lemon and Thyme OR Use any White fish
Ingredients:

32 oz piece of salmon or any fresh white fish

1 lemon, sliced thin

1 tbsp capers

low sodium salt and freshly ground pepper

1 tbsp fresh thyme

Olive oil

Instructions:

Line a rimmed baking sheet with parchment paper and place salmon, skin side down, on the prepared baking sheet.

Season salmon with low sodium salt and pepper. Arrange capers on the salmon, and top with sliced lemon and thyme.

Place baking sheet in a cold oven, then turn heat to 400 degrees F. Bake for 25 minutes. Serve immediately.

86. Spectacular Shrimp Scampi in Spaghetti Sauce
Ingredients:

For the Spaghetti:

1 spaghetti squash

Extra virgin olive oil, for drizzling

low sodium salt and pepper

1 tsp dried oregano

1 tsp dried basil

For the shrimp scampi:

8 oz. shrimp, peeled and deveined

3 tbsp butter

1 tbsp extra virgin olive oil

2 cloves garlic, minced

Pinch of red pepper flakes

low sodium salt and pepper, to taste

1 tbsp fresh parsley, chopped

Juice of 1 lemon

Zest of half a lemon

Instructions:

Preheat the oven to 400 degrees F. Place squash in the microwave for 3-4 minutes to soften. Using a sharp knife, cut the squash in half lengthwise. Scoop out the seeds and discard. Place the halves, with the cut side up, on a rimmed baking sheet.

Drizzle with olive oil and sprinkle with seasonings. Roast in the oven for 45-50 minutes, until you can poke the squash easily with a fork.

Let it cool until you can handle it safely. Then scrape the insides with a fork to shred the squash into strands.

After removing spaghetti squash from the oven, melt the butter and olive oil in a skillet over medium heat.

Add in the garlic and sauté for 2-3 minutes. Then add in the shrimp, low sodium salt, pepper, and a pinch of red pepper flakes.

Cook for 5 minutes, until the shrimp is cooked through. Remove from heat and add in desired amount of cooked spaghetti squash. Toss with lemon juice and zest. Top with parsley.

87. Scrumptious Cod in Delish Sauce

Ingredients:

1 lb. cod fillets

1/3 cup almond flour

1/2 tsp low sodium salt

2-3 tbsp extra virgin olive oil

2 tbsp walnut oil, divided

3/4 cup low sodium chicken stock

3 tbsp lemon juice

1/4 cup capers, drained

2 tbsp fresh parsley, chopped

Instructions:

Stir the almond flour and low sodium salt together in a shallow bowl. Rinse off the fish and pat dry with a paper towel. Dredge the fish in the almond flour mixture to coat.

Heat enough olive oil to coat the bottom of a large skillet over medium-high heat along with one tablespoon walnut oil. Working in batches, add the cod and cook for 2-3 minutes per side to brown. Remove to a plate and set aside.

Add the chicken stock, lemon juice, and capers to the same skillet and scrape any browned bits off the bottom. Simmer to reduce the sauce by almost half. Remove from heat and stir in the remaining tablespoon of walnut oil.

To serve, divide the cod onto plates, drizzle with the sauce, and sprinkle with parsley.

88. Delish Baked dill Salmon

Ingredients:

2 6-oz. salmon fillets

2 zucchini, halved lengthwise and thinly sliced

1/4 red onion, thinly sliced

1 tsp fresh dill, chopped

2 slices lemon

1 tbsp fresh lemon juice

Extra virgin olive oil, for drizzling

low sodium salt and freshly

ground pepper

Instructions:

Preheat the oven to 350 degrees F. Prepare a baking tray

Place half of the zucchini, red onion, dill, and one lemon slice. Drizzle with olive oil and sprinkle with low sodium salt and pepper. Place a salmon fillet on top and drizzle with the lemon juice. Season with low sodium salt and pepper. Repeat with the remaining ingredients.

Bake for 15-20 minutes until the salmon is opaque.

89. Prawn garlic Fried "Rice"

Ingredients:

1 tbsp coconut oil

1 cup white onion, finely chopped

2 cloves garlic, minced

8 oz. prawns peeled and deveined

1 medium carrot, chopped

1/2 cup peas

2 cups cooked cauliflower rice

2 eggs, beaten

Low sodium salt and pepper, to taste

Instructions:

Heat a wok or large pan over medium-high heat. Melt the coconut oil and add the onion and garlic to the pan.

Cook for 3-4 minutes until the onion starts to soften. Add the shrimp and cook for 1 minute.

Add the carrot, peas, and bell pepper to the pan. Cook for 3-4 minutes, and then stir in the cauliflower rice.

Clear a circle in the center of the pan and pour in the beaten eggs. Stir to scramble the eggs and then combine with the other ingredients.

Season with low sodium salt and pepper to taste.

90. Lemon and Thyme Super Salmon

Ingredients:

32 oz piece of salmon

1 lemon, sliced thin

2 tspns lemon juice

Low sodium salt and freshly ground pepper

1 tbsp fresh thyme

Olive oil, for drizzling

Instructions:

Wrap all ingredients into tin foil and place inside a preheated hot oven (350 deg) for 15 minutes

Season with low sodium salt and pepper to taste.

91. Delicious Salmon in Herb Crust

Ingredients:

2 salmon fillets (approx. 300g)

1 small onion, peeled and quartered

2 garlic cloves, peeled

1 sprig lemongrass, coarsely chopped

2 cm piece of ginger root, peeled

1 red chili pepper

Instructions:

Line a rimmed baking sheet with parchment paper and place salmon, skin side down, on the prepared baking sheet.

Generously season salmon with low sodium salt and pepper and top with sliced lemon and thyme.

Place baking sheet in a cold oven, then turn heat to 400 degrees F. Bake for 25 minutes.

Add lemon juice and serve immediately.

92. Salmon Mustard Delish
Ingredients:

4 tsp mustard seed

1/2 tsp garlic powder

1/4 tsp low sodium salt

1/4 tsp black pepper

1/4 tsp dried dill

1 1/2 lb salmon

Instructions:

Preheat oven to 200 degrees Celsius. (390 F)

Start by making the herb crust: combine all the ingredients in the smallest bowl of a food processor

Process into a coarse paste.

Put the salmon fillets in an oven dish and spread the herb paste on top.

Bake for approx. 12-15 minutes until done, depending on the thickness of your fillets.

Serve with veggies of your choice and enjoy!

93. Sexy Spicy Salmon
Ingredients:

For the Salmon:

4 6 ounce Sockeye Salmon Filets

½ teaspoon of Cinnamon

½ teaspoon of Coriander

½ teaspoon of Cumin

¼ teaspoon of Ground Cloves

¼ teaspoon of Cardamom

low sodium salt to taste

1 Tablespoon of coconut butter

For the Lime Mustard dressing:

¼ cup of olive oil

1 Tablespoon of Lime Juice

2 teaspoons of mustard powder

Pinch of low sodium salt

Instructions:

Preheat the oven to 425°F. Grind all of the spices together with a mortar and pestle until most are powder, and everything is well blended.

Spread the mixture over the salmon evenly, and place on a baking pan with a non-stick rack.

Bake for 15 to 20 minutes, until the flesh flakes easily with a fork. If you prefer salmon that is medium-rare, 15 minutes should do the trick.

Enjoy the dressing with your favorite sautéed greens, or mixed salad.

94. Mouthwatering Stuffed Salmon
Ingredients:

1 lb wild Alaskan or sockeye salmon, cut into 2 pieces

6 oz raw shrimp, peeled, deveined and chopped

1 large egg

2 tbsp raw onions, chopped

2 tbsp Italian flat leaf parsley, chopped

2 tbsp almond meal (or almond flour)

2 tbsp coconut butter

1 clove garlic, minced

low sodium salt and pepper to taste

Instructions:

For the Salmon:

Preheat oven to 400F

Pat dry the salmon filets with a paper towel.

Combine the cinnamon, coriander, cumin, cloves, and cardamom. Sprinkle evenly over the salmon filet side.

Heat an oven safe skillet (preferably cast iron) to medium high heat. Test the heat by placing a drop of water. It should immediately evaporate.

Add the coconut butter and let it melt.

Place the salmon filet side down and let sear for about 1-2 minutes. Flip and sear on the skin side for 1 minute.

Place the skillet inside the oven, with the skin side down.

Bake at 400F for 6-7 minutes.

For the Lime Mustard Mayo:

Combine dressing, lime juice, low sodium salt, and mustard.

Dip with salmon and enjoy!

95. Spectacular Salmon

Ingredients:

For the salmon:

2 salmon fillets (6oz each)

1 heaping tablespoon coconut flour

2 tablespoons fresh parsley

1 tablespoon olive oil

1 tablespoon mustard powder

low sodium salt and pepper, to taste

For the salad:

2 cups any green leaf salad

¼ red onion, sliced thin

juice of 1 lemon

1 tablespoon white wine vinegar

1 tablespoon olive oil

low sodium salt and pepper, to taste

Instructions:

Preheat oven to 375F.

Mix the chopped raw shrimp, egg, onions, parsley, almond meal, 1tbsp coconut butter, garlic, low sodium salt and pepper. Set aside.

Lightly season the salmon pieces with low sodium salt and pepper. Heat a cast iron pan on high and add the rest of the lard. Pan sear the salmon 1-2 minutes per side.

Move the salmon to an ovenproof dish and top each piece with 2 tbsp (or more!) of the shrimp topping. Lightly brush the top with a little bit of lard and bake in the oven for 15 minutes.

Afterwards, set your oven to broil and cook for about 3 more minutes until the top becomes crispy.

96. Creamy Coconut Salmon

Ingredients:

1 pound wild salmon fillets

¼ tsp low sodium salt

¼ tsp freshly ground black pepper

2 tsp coconut oil

3 cloves fresh garlic (minced)

1 large shallot (minced)

1 lemon (juice and zest)

½ cup unsweetened full-fat coconut milk

Instructions:

Preheat oven to 450 degrees.

Place salmon fillets on a parchment or foil lined baking sheet.

Top your salmon off with olive oil and mustard powder and rub into your salmon.

In a small bowl, mix together your coconut flour, parsley, and low sodium salt and pepper.

Use a spoon to sprinkle on your toppings on your salmon and then your hand to pat into your salmon.

Place in oven for 10-15 minutes or until salmon is cooked to your preference. I cooked mine more on the medium rare side at 12 minutes.

While the salmon is cooking, mix together your salad ingredients.

When salmon is done, place salmon on top of salad and consume.

97. Salmon Dill Bonanza

Ingredients:

1 1/2 pounds wild salmon (I used sockeye)

zest of one lemon (about a tablespoon)

2 tablespoons oil

1 tablespoon chopped, fresh dill

1 lemon

low sodium salt and pepper

Instructions:

Preheat oven to 375°F.

Place salmon in a shallow baking dish and season with low sodium salt and pepper.

Heat coconut oil in a medium saute pan or cast iron skillet over medium heat. Add garlic and shallots and saute until tender and fragrant, 3-5 minutes.

Add lemon zest, lemon juice, and coconut milk, stirring to combine.

Bring to a low boil, then remove from heat.

Pour mixture over salmon. Bake, uncovered, for 10-20 minutes or until salmon flakes easily with a fork.

98. Sexy Shrimp Cocktail

Ingredients:

1 pound uncooked shrimp, peeled, deveined, and thawed if frozen

1 tablespoon olive oil

Low sodium salt and fresh ground pepper to taste

1 cup coconut cream and two tablespoon tomato paste

One teaspoon fresh pressed garlic

lemon wedges

Instructions:

Preheat oven to 400 degrees F.

Oil the bottom of a 9 x 13 baking dish.

Rinse the salmon and pat dry with paper towels. Sprinkle with low sodium salt and pepper and place in the prepared dish.

Mix together the oil (room temperature), lemon zest and dill.

Place about half the mixture on top of the seasoned salmon. You can spread the lemon dill mixture or leave it in dollops like this.

Bake for about 10-15 minutes. The salmon will continue cooking even after you take it out of the oven.

Add the remaining oil/dill/lemon zest mixture on top, add a squeeze of lemon juice.

99. Gambas al Ajillo--Sizzling Garlic Shrimp

Ingredients:

1/2 cup olive oil

10 cloves garlic, peeled and thinly sliced

1 pound raw shrimp, peeled, deveined, and tails removed, defrosted if frozen

Low sodium salt and pepper to taste

1/4 teaspoon paprika

Pinch or two of red pepper flakes, optional

Instructions:

Preheat oven to 425 degrees.

Toss shrimp with oil, low sodium salt and pepper and spread in single layer on rimmed baking sheet.

Roast, turning once, until shrimp is pink and just cooked through (about 5-10 minutes, depending on size of shrimp).

Serve chilled with the blend of coconut cream, tomato paste and pressed garlic...add black pepper and lemon wedges.

100. Garlic Lemon Shrimp Bonanza

Ingredients:

1 lb shrimp, deveined

3-4 cloves of garlic, chopped

1/2 fresh lemon juice

3 tbsp olive oil

1/8 of low sodium salt

Fresh ground pepper (to taste)

1 tbsp fresh parsley, chopped for garnish

Instructions:

Preheat the broiler, if using. Heat the olive oil in a heavy skillet over medium-low heat.

Add the garlic and saute, stirring frequently, for about five minutes, until the garlic is softened but not browned.

Add the shrimp, raise the heat to medium high, and sprinkle with low sodium salt, pepper, paprika, and red pepper.

Cook for three minutes on each side or until the shrimp are completely opaque. Serve hot.

101. Courgette Pesto and Shrimp

Ingredients:

For the Pesto Sauce:

A ton of Basil

Minced Garlic

Pine Nuts

low sodium salt & Pepper

For the Zinguine:

1 Small Zucchini

low sodium salt & Pepper to taste

For the Shrimp:

Shrimp (peeled & de-veined)

Instructions:

Heat pan to medium-high heat.

Add ghee and garlic. Saute for about a minute.

Add shrimp. Saute for about a minute on each side.

Add low sodium salt, pepper and lemon juice. Saute for another minute or so.

Remove from heat and dish onto a plate or bowl.

102. Easy Shrimp Stir Fry

Ingredients:

1lb of wild shrimp

1 Lemon

3 Cloves of garlic, minced

2 Tablespoons of olive oil

1/2 teaspoon of garlic power

1 Dash of red pepper flakes

4 Tablespoons of olive oil

Instructions:

Throw all ingredients in a mini food processor. Pulse until it's a paste that you think looks and smells delicious.

Use a vegetable peeler and peel the courgette right into the pan, then saute.

Stir in pesto sauce and low sodium salt /pepper when the zucchini linguine starts turning transparent.

In another smaller skillet, cook shrimp over medium heat for approximately 3 minutes per side.

103. Delectable Shrimp Scampi

Ingredients:

4 tsp olive oil

1 1/4 pounds med raw shrimp, peeled and deveined (tails left on)

6-8 garlic cloves, minced

1/2 cup low sodium chicken broth

1/4 cup fresh lemon juice

1/4 cup + 1 T minced parsley

1/4 tsp low sodium salt

1/4 tsp freshly ground pepper

4 lemon wedges

Instructions:

Peal shrimp and butterfly them (making a cut in the back and extracting the vein).

Place shrimp in marinade: 2 Tablespoons olive oil, lemon, garlic powder. Marinade anywhere from 15 minutes to hours (the more time, the better)

Heat 2 Tablespoons of oil in pan on medium to high heat.

Add shrimp and cook each side for 2-3 minutes. Drizzle with 1 Tablespoon of olive oil.

Top with low sodium salt, pepper, and red pepper flakes.

104. Citrus Shrimp Delux
Ingredients:

3/4 pounds peeled and deveined medium-large shrimp

1/2 Tbls almond meal

2 Tbls orange juice, fresh squeezed

1/2 Tbls rice vinegar

1 Tbls diced chillies

1 Tbls olive oil

1/2 Tbls fresh ginger, minced

2 garlic cloves, minced

Instructions:

In a large nonstick skillet, heat the oil. Saute the shrimp until just pink, about 2-3 minutes. Add the garlic and cook stirring constantly, about 30 seconds. With a slotted spoon transfer the shrimp to a platter and keep them warm.

In the skillet, combine the broth, lemon juice, 1/4 cup of the parsley, the low sodium salt and pepper; and bring it to a boil. Boil uncovered, until the sauce is reduced by half.

Spoon the sauce over the shrimp. Serve garnished with the lemon wedges and sprinkled with the remaining tablespoon of parsley.

105. Sexy Garlic Shrimp

Ingredients:

4-5 T olive oil

4 garlic cloves, minced

1 t red pepper flakes

1 t smoked paprika

1 lb medium shrimp, peeled and deveined

2 T fresh lime juice

2 Teaspoons jerez sherry

low sodium salt and pepper to taste

drop stevia

Instructions:

Place shrimp in bowl and toss with almond powder.

 Make sure shrimp is evenly coated.

In a small bowl whisk together orange juice, stevia, rice vinegar and chili

Heat olive oil in a large non-stick skillet over medium-high heat. Add ginger and garlic. Stir until garlic becomes fragrant. This will only take 10-15 seconds.

Add shrimp and cook for 3 minutes. Add in sauce and cook for additional 2 minutes. Remove shrimp with a slotted spoon.

Continue stirring sauce for another 2-4 minutes until it thickens. Drizzle over shrimp. Serve on top of baby spinach or fried cauliflower rice.

106. Shrimp Cakes Delux

Ingredients:

2 cups of small prawns

2 eggs

fresh chives

1/2 tsp spicy chili powder

1/2 tsp ground coriander

1/2 tsp garlic powder

shredded coconut

1/2 tbsp coconut flour

Instructions:

In a saute pan over medium heat, warm the olive oil.

Add the garlic, red pepper flakes and paprika and saute for 1 minute until fragrant.

Increase the heat to high, add the shrimp, lime juice and sherry, stir well, and saute until the shrimp.

Season with low sodium salt and black pepper.

107. Shrimp Spinach Spectacular
Ingredients:

2 tablespoons olive oil

½ yellow onion – diced

1 cup green beans

2 cloves garlic minced

½ teaspoon chili powder

½ lime – juiced

1 pound raw wild shrimp – thawed, cleaned, and tails removed

1 – 6 oz. bag of baby spinach

low sodium salt and pepper to taste

Instructions:

Heat the oil and add everything except the shrimp, beans and spinach.

Add the green beans first and simmer until softened

Add the shrimp keeping heat high and simmer for just a few seconds

Add the spinach and stir in for another 20 seconds

Ate up and In a large sauté pan, heat olive oil over medium heat. Add onion, beans, and sauté until tender – approximately 10 minutes.

Add garlic, lime juice, and chili powder and continue to cook for an additional 5 minutes.

Add spinach and shrimp. Continue to cook for approximately 7-10 more minutes until spinach has wilted and shrimp is done.

 Enjoy immediately – optional lime juice can be squeezed over

108. Prawn Salad Boats

Ingredients:

1 lb shrimp, cooked

1 medium tomato, diced

1 cucumber, peeled and diced

 3 tablespoons olive oil

One tablespoon coconut cream

Juice of one lemon

1/2 tsp dried dill

1/2 tsp celery seed

1/4 tsp low sodium salt

1/4 tsp pepper

Endive or big lettuce leaf, for serving

Instructions:

In a medium bowl, mix the coconut cream, and lemon juice until combined.

Add the shrimp, tomato, cucumbers, capers, and spices.

Mix until everything is incorporated. Add additional low sodium salt and pepper to taste. Serve in endive leaves.

109. Cheeky Curry Shrimp

Ingredients:

1 lb raw, peeled, tail on shrimp

2 tsp curry powder

1 tsp garlic powder

1 tsp ground coriander

1/2 tsp ground ginger

low sodium salt and black pepper to taste

Instructions:

Rinse shrimp under cold water and pat dry with a paper towel.

Place shrimp in a large Ziploc bag.

In a small mixing bowl, curry powder, coriander, garlic powder, ground ginger, low sodium salt, and pepper.

Pour spice mixture over shrimp, seal bag, and toss to evenly coat.

Place shrimp in the fridge and allow to marinate for at least an hour.

Preheat grill to high heat.

Grill shrimp about 6 minutes

Serve alongside your choice of vegetable or fried cauliflower rice.

110. Courgette Shrimp Coquettes

Ingredients:

1 pound fresh shrimp, peeled and deveined

4-5 medium courgettes julienned very small, about the size of spaghetti

1 onion, chopped

2 cloves garlic, chopped

1 can diced tomatoes, with liquid (14 oz.)

2 cups fresh spinach

1/2 tsp red chili flake

1 tsp fresh oregano

1 tbsp fresh lemon juice

1 tbsp olive oil

Instructions:

Heat olive oil in a large pan over medium heat. Add onion and garlic and cook until tender. Add chili flake and stir for about a minute.

When that has cooked down, add the diced tomatoes and oregano. Simmer for about 10 minutes.

Add julienned zucchini and lemon juice and cook, stirring, for about 5 minutes.

Add shrimp and then the spinach, once shrimp is just cooked through. Low sodium salt and pepper to taste and serve with a fresh squeeze of lemon.

111. Sexy Shrimp on Sticks

Ingredients:

1/2 lb shrimp, peeled and deveined

1/4 cup coconut milk

1 tsp fish sauce

6 gloves garlic, chopped

1/4 tsp each turmeric, cumin, low sodium salt

Instructions:

Thread the shrimp onto a thin wooden stick suitable for grilling

Marinate for at least an hour or longer in the rest of the ingredients

Grill at 200 degrees for 10 minutes each side

Serve with a mixed salad of choice

112. Delicious Fish Stir Fry
Ingredients:

200 grams any white fish fillet (cut into pieces)

1 Tablespoon Coconut Vinegar

1/2 Teaspoon Ginger and Garlic fresh pressed

1 small onion (quartered)

1/2 Cup Bell Peppers de-seeded and cubed (Red or Yellow).

1/2 Cup Mushrooms (any kind)

2 to 3 stalks of scallions (cut into 1.5 inch length)

low sodium salt to taste

1 Teaspoon Chili powder (Optional)

1 Teaspoon Fish Sauce

1/2 Tablespoon Extra Virgin Olive Oil

Instructions:

In a large bowl mix fish sauce, garlic and ginger.

Heat the olive oil in a wok (or a large nonstick skillet) over medium-high heat.

Once it starts to shimmer add ginger and garlic until they start to brown around the edges, about 2 minutes.

Stir in the other vegetables and chilli powder and stir-fry for 1 minute.

Add the fish sauce and cook until it's nearly cooked through about 2 minutes, stirring often.

Add coconut vinegar and stir-fry for 30 seconds or so, until the greens are wilted. Serve immediately.

113. Sexy Shrimp with Delish Veggie Stir Fry

Ingredients:

1 1/2 pounds of shrimp

2 tbsn. of coconut oil

1/2 cup of thinly sliced garlic, ginger and green onion

1/2 red bell pepper and 2 carrots. thinly sliced

1 cup of full fat coconut milk

2 tbsp. fish sauce

1 tbsp curry powder

2 tbsp. of chopped cilantro

sesame oil

Instructions:

Heat 2 tbsp. coconut oil in a wok or large pan.

Add the sliced garlic and grated ginger to the wok and stir-fry for 30 seconds.

Add the green onion, fish sauce and curry powder and stir-fry 1 more minute.

Add the bell pepper and carrot and stir-fry about a minute. You want it just barely cooked, not limp and soggy.

Stir-fry until just done and no more. To check, I like to cut open the biggest piece to make sure it isn't pink in the middle.

Add the sesame oil.

114. Sexy Spicy Salmon

Ingredients:

Stevia to taste

1 1/2 lemons, juice of

1/2 tsp garlic powder

3 tbsp soy sauce, reduced sodium gluten free

14 oz wild salmon fillets, cut into 4 pieces

1 clove crushed garlic

1 tbsp chilli flakes

7 oz sliced shiitake mushrooms

1 tbsp fresh ginger, finely minced

1 cup snap peas

1/2 cup sliced scallions, divided

1 tbsp black sesame seeds

Instructions:

Mix stevia, juice of half a lemon, garlic powder, and 1 tbsp of the soy sauce in bowl. Add salmon to marinade and set aside in refrigerator up to 30 minutes turning once after 15 minutes; reserve the marinade.

Add the remaining ingredients: 2 tbsp soy sauce, remaining lemon juice, crushed garlic, and chilli flakes. Add mushrooms, ginger, snap peas, 1/4 cup scallions and cook on medium heat for 5 minutes.

Meanwhile, heat a nonstick skillet on medium heat sprayed lightly with cooking spray, remove salmon from marinade but do not discard, cook salmon 2 minutes on each side then add the marinade, cover and cook on low heat 5 minutes. Serve the vegetables in a dish and top with salmon, remaining scallions and sesame seeds.

Serve with cauliflower rice.

115. Delish Skewered Shrimp

Ingredients:

Wooden skewers, soaked in water for 30 minutes

1-1/2 lbs large shrimp, peeled and deveined

Chilli flakes, garlic flakes, onion powder to taste

Instructions:

Preheat the grill. Thread shrimp onto skewers and season

Cook shrimp over medium/hot flame. When shrimp start to turn pink … turn. Repeat every 3 to 4 minutes until done. Serve hot and enjoy!

Serve with a green salad

116. Lemon Tilapia Ajillo

Ingredients:

6 (6 oz each) tilapia filets

4 cloves garlic, crushed

2 tbsp olive oil

2 tbsp fresh lemon juice

4 tsp fresh parsley

Low sodium salt and pepper

cooking spray

large romaine lettuce, 1 grated carrot, half grated onion, handful baby tomatoes

Basic Paleo Dressing:

2 tblspoon best quality olive oil

1 tbspn apple cider vinegar

Squirt of fresh lemon juice

Half teaspoon garlic powder and half teaspoon onion powder

Black pepper to taste

Instructions:

Preheat oven to 400°.

Melt butter on a low flame in a small sauce pan. Add garlic and saute on low for about 1 minute. Add the lemon juice and shut off flame.

Spray the bottom of a baking dish lightly with cooking spray. Place the fish on top and season with low sodium salt and pepper. Pour the lemon butter mixture on the fish and top with fresh parsley. Bake at 400° until cooked, about 15 minutes.

Serve with a mixed salad and paleo dressing

117. Tantalizing Prawn Skewers
Ingredients:

1 lb jumbo raw tiger prawns, shelled and deveined (weight after peeled)

2 cloves garlic, crushed

Low sodium salt and pepper

8 long wooden skewers

Instructions:

Soak the skewers in water at least 20 minutes to prevent them from burning.

Combine the prawns with crushed garlic and season with low sodium salt and pepper. You can let this marinate for a while, or even overnight.

Heat a clean, lightly oiled grill to medium heat, when the grill is hot add the prawns, careful not to burn the skewers. Grill on both sides for about 6 - 8 minutes total cooking time or until the prawns are opaque and cooked through.

Squeeze lemon juice over the prawns and serve with green salad and my paleo dressing

118. Seared Salmon with Mango Salsa

Ingredients:

For the mango salsa:

1 large ripe mango peeled, seeded and coarsely chopped

1-2 tbsp chopped fresh cilantro

1 small clove garlic, minced

2 tbsp fresh lime juice

For the salmon:

1 tablespoon paprika

1 tablespoon cayenne

5 sprigs fresh thyme, washed, leaves removed and chopped

1 tablespoon freshly chopped oregano leaves

1 teaspoon low sodium salt

1 lb (4 pieces) wild salmon fillet, skin-on

cooking spray ….always use olive oil not canola

Instructions:

Combine all the salsa ingredients in a bowl, season to taste with low sodium salt and pepper and refrigerate salsa until ready to serve. Makes 1 cup.

In a small bowl, add the paprika, cayenne, thyme and oregano and low sodium salt and mix to blend. Put the mixture on a plate or other flat surface and coat the salmon fillets.

Heat a large heavy-bottomed pan or cast iron skillet over medium heat, and generously spray with oil. When very hot add the salmon, flesh side down and cook for 2 to 3 minutes. Use a spatula to carefully turn the salmon, then cook an additional 5 to 6 minutes.

Arrange the salmon on a platter, top with salsa and serve immediately with a green salad

119. Sexy Rosemary Salmon
Ingredients:

24 oz or 4 pieces of salmon

olive oil spray

2 tsp fresh lemon juice

2 tsp fresh, chopped rosemary

2 cloves garlic, minced

Low sodium salt and fresh pepper to taste

Instructions:

Combine lemon juice, rosemary, low sodium salt, pepper and garlic. Brush mixture onto fish.

Spray a ridged frying pan with olive oil spray and arrange the fish on it.

Cook to level of preferred inner pinkness!...and turn of course

120. Broiled Curry Coconut Sole or Cod
Ingredients:

1 tsp dark sesame oil, divided

1 tbsp minced peeled fresh ginger

4 garlic cloves, minced

1 cup finely chopped red bell pepper

1 cup chopped scallions

1 tsp curry powder

2 tsp red curry paste

1/2 tsp ground cumin

4 tsp low-sodium soy sauce

Stevia to taste

1 (14-ounce) can light coconut milk

1/4 cup chopped fresh cilantro

6 (6-ounce) fish fillets

Low sodium salt

Cooking spray

Instructions:

Preheat broiler.

Heat 1/2 teaspoon oil in a large nonstick skillet over medium heat. Add ginger and garlic; cook 1 minute. Add pepper and scallions; cook 1 minute. Stir in curry powder, curry paste, and cumin; cook 1 minute. Add soy sauce, stevia, and coconut milk; bring to a simmer (do not boil). Remove from heat; stir in cilantro or basil if using.

Brush fish with 1/2 teaspoon oil; sprinkle with 1/4 teaspoon low sodium salt. Place fish on a baking sheet coated with cooking spray. Broil 7 minutes or until fish flakes easily when tested with a fork. Serve fish with sauce and lime wedges.

Serve with cauliflower rice

121. Oregano Prawns

Ingredients:

1 tbsp finely chopped fresh oregano or 1 tsp dried

10 tiger prawns

1/2 tsp low sodium salt

1/4 tsp fresh pepper

4 tsp olive oil

1 garlic clove, minced

Instructions:

Preheat broiler. Line broiling pan with aluminum foil.

Add prawns Season with low sodium salt, pepper and oregano. Add garlic, drizzle with oil.

Arrange fillets in a single layer on the prepared pan. Broil about 8 inches from the heat until the topping is browned. Be careful not to overcook

Serve with lime and your favorite vegetables.

122. Tasty Tomato Tilapia

Ingredients:

2 tbsp extra virgin olive oil

4 (6 oz) tilapia filets

2 garlic cloves, crushed

2 shallots, minced

2 tomatoes, chopped

2 tbsp capers

1/4 cup white wine

Low sodium salt and fresh pepper

Instructions:

Brush fish with 1 tbsp olive and season with low sodium salt and pepper.

In a medium sauté pan, heat remaining olive oil. Add garlic and shallots and sauté on medium-low about 4-5 minutes. Add tomatoes and season with low sodium salt and pepper. Add wine and sauté until wine reduces, about 5 minutes. Add capers and sauté an additional minute.

Meanwhile, set broiler to low and place fish about 8 inches from the flame. Broil until fish is cooked through, about 7 minutes.

Place fish on a platter and top with tomato caper sauce.

Eat with a green salad and paleo dressing

123. Prawn Asparagus Stir Fry

Ingredients:

2 tbsp low sodium soy sauce (use tamari for gluten free)

1 tsp sherry

1 tbsp grated peeled fresh ginger

2 tsp sesame oil

1 pound asparagus, trimmed and cut diagonally into 2-inch pieces

1 chili pepper, sliced

2 cloves garlic, chopped

1 bell pepper, sliced

1 lb large tiger prawns, cleaned

Low sodium salt and pepper to taste

Instructions:

Stir together soy sauce, sherry and ginger; set aside.

In a wok, heat 1 tsp sesame oil over medium-high heat until hot. Add prawns and cook until white, about 3 minutes. Remove from wok and set aside.

Add remaining oil to wok. When oil is hot, add asparagus and cook 5 minutes or until tender-crisp, stirring frequently. Add garlic. Add peppers and stir another minute. Add prawns back into the wok. Pour sauce over everything and mix another minute. Adjust low sodium salt and pepper to taste.

Serve with cauliflower rice

124. Cilantro Fish Delish

Ingredients:

1 1/2 pounds fresh cod or any white fish

1/4 teaspoon plus 1/8 teaspoon ground cumin

Low sodium salt and freshly ground black pepper

2 teaspoons extra-virgin olive oil

5 garlic cloves, crushed

2 tablespoons lime juice (from 1 medium lime)

3 to 4 tablespoons chopped fresh cilantro

Instructions:

Season the fish with cumin, and low sodium salt and pepper to taste.

Heat a large nonstick skillet over medium-high heat. Add 1 teaspoon of the oil to the pan, then add half of the fish. Cook them undisturbed for about 2 minutes. Turn the shrimp over and cook until opaque throughout, about 1 minute. Transfer to a plate.

Add the remaining 1 teaspoon oil and the remaining fish to the pan and cook, undisturbed, for about 2 minutes. Turn the shrimp over, add the garlic, and cook until the shrimp is opaque throughout, about 1 minute. Return the first batch to the skillet, mix well so that the garlic is evenly incorporated and remove the pan from the heat.

Squeeze the lime juice over all the shrimp. Add the cilantro, toss well, and serve with cauliflower rice

125. Perfect Prawns

Ingredients:

2 tsp extra virgin olive oil

1.25 lb large or jumbo prawns, peeled and deveined (1 lb after peeled)

6 garlic cloves, chopped

1 tsp crushed red pepper flakes

fresh pepper to taste

2 tablespoons of capers (rinsed)

1/4 cup of white wine

1 cup clam juice

juice from one lemon

generous handful of chopped parsley

celeriac mash see below

Instructions:

Heat olive oil in a skillet. Add garlic, pepper flakes, and sauté 2-3 minutes.

Add wine, clam juice, lemon juice, parsley, low sodium salt and pepper, and stir. Cook for another 2-3 minutes.

Add prawns and cook for 2-3 minutes. Do not overcook or it will become tough and chewy. Serve with liquid in a bowl and some celeriac mash (boil 3 cups diced celeriac for 10 minutes and blend with olive oil and garlic powder)

126. Fish Fillet Delux
Ingredients:

4 white fish fillets, about 5 oz each

4 tsp olive oil

Low sodium salt and fresh pepper, to taste

4 sprigs fresh herbs (parsley, rosemary, oregano)

1 lemon, sliced thin

4 large pieces heavy duty aluminum foil,

Instructions:

Place the fish in the center of the foil, season with low sodium salt and pepper and drizzle with olive oil. Place a slice of lemon on top of each piece of fish, then a sprig of herbs on each. Fold up the edges so that it's completely sealed and no steam will escape, creating a loose tent.

Heat half of the grill (on one side) on high heat with the cover closed. When the grill is hot, place the foil packets on the side of the grill with the burners off (indirect heat) and close the grill. Depending on the thickness of your fish, cook 10 to 15 minutes, or until the fish is opaque and cooked through.....serve with green salad and paleo dressing.

127. Gambas Ajillo

Ingredients:

1 lb large shrimp, peeled and deveined (weight after you peel them)

6 cloves garlic, sliced thin

1 tbsp Spanish olive oil

crushed red pepper flakes

pinch paprika

low sodium salt

Instructions:

In a large skillet, heat oil on medium heat and add the garlic and red pepper flakes. Sauté until golden, about 2 minutes being careful not to burn.

Add shrimp and season with salt and paprika. Cook 2-3 minutes until shrimp is cooked through. Do not overcook or it will become tough and chewy.

See previous recipe for celeriac mash!

128. Peachy Prawn Coconut

Ingredients:

1 1/4 lbs jumbo prawns, peeled and deveined (weight after peeled)

1 tsp extra virgin olive oil

1 red bell pepper, sliced thin

4 scallions, thinly sliced, white and green parts separated

1/2 cup cilantro

4 cloves garlic, minced

Low sodium salt (to taste)

1/2 tsp crushed red pepper flakes (to taste)

14.5 oz can diced tomatoes

14 oz can light coconut milk (50% less fat)*

1/2 lime, squeezed

Instructions:

In a medium pot, heat oil on low. Add red peppers and sauté until soft (about 4 minutes). Add scallion whites, 1/4 cup cilantro, red pepper flakes and garlic. Cook 1 minute.

Add tomatoes, coconut milk and low sodium salt to taste, cover and simmer on low about 10 minutes to let the flavors blend together and to thicken the sauce.

Add prawns and cook 5 minutes. Add lime juice.

To serve, divide equally among 4 bowls and top with scallions and cilantro.

Serve with cauliflower rice

129. Highly Delish Herb Salmon

Ingredients:

4 garlic cloves

1 tsp dried Herbs de Provence

1 tsp red wine vinegar

1 tsp olive oil

2 tbsp mustard powder

olive oil spray

4 (6 oz) wild salmon fillets, 1" thick (if frozen, thaw first)

Low sodium salt and fresh ground pepper to taste

4 lemon wedges for serving

Instructions:

In a mini food processor, or using a mortar and pestle mash garlic with the herbs, vinegar, oil, and mustard until it becomes a paste. Set aside.

Season salmon with a pinch of low sodium salt and fresh pepper. Heat a grill or grill pan over high heat until hot. Spray the pan lightly with oil and reduce the heat to medium-low. Place the salmon on the hot grill pan and cook without moving for 5 minutes.

Turn and cook the other side for an additional 3-4 minutes spooning on half of the garlic herb mustard sauce.

Turn and cook 1 more minute spooning the other side of the fish with remaining sauce. Turn once again and let the fish finish cooking about one more minute.

Serve with a green salad and paleo dressing

130. Happy Halibut Soup

Ingredients:

1 tsp olive oil

2 chopped shallots

2 cloves of garlic

3 medium diced tomatoes

4 oz cup of white wine

1 cup clam juice

2 cups vegetable stock

3/4 lb halibut filet, skin removed cut into large pieces

1 dozen small clams

pinch of saffron

1/4 cup fresh chopped parsley

Instructions:

Add olive oil to a large heavy pot; over medium heat sautée shallots and garlic until translucent. Add the tomatoes, wine, clam juice and the bone from the halibut if you have one. Add vegetable stock, saffron, fresh thyme and stir.

Add the clams; cover and cook 2 minutes, add the fish and cook and additional 3 minutes, or until the shrimp turns pink and the clams open.

131. Tasty Teriyaki Salmon

Ingredients:

3 tbsp low-sodium soy sauce (or tamari for gluten free)

3 tbsp mirin (Japanese sweet rice wine)

3 tbsp sake

Stevia to taste

1 lb fresh wild salmon fillet, cut in 4 pieces

2 tsp cooking oil

Instructions:

Combine the soy sauce, mirin, sake, and stevia in a resealable bag.

Add the salmon and mix to coat. Refrigerate for 1 hour or up to 8 hours.

Remove salmon, reserving the marinade. Heat a frying pan or sauté pan over medium-high heat. When hot, swirl in the oil.

Sear salmon, 2 minutes per side. Turn heat to low and pour in the reserved marinade. Cover and cook for 4 to 5 minutes, until cooked through.

Serve with cauliflower rice

132. Sexy Shrimp Cakes

Ingredients:

1 lb shrimp, peeled and deveined (weight after peeled)

1 large jalapeño, seeded and minced (for spicy, leave the seeds)

1 garlic clove, minced

3 medium scallions, chopped

2 tablespoons fresh cilantro, chopped

1/4 teaspoon low sodium salt

1/8 teaspoon fresh ground black pepper

1 tablespoon almond flour for binding

For topping:

4 lime wedges

1/2 medium avocado, sliced thin

Instructions:

Dry shrimp well with a paper towel then place the shrimp in the food processor along with jalapeño and garlic then pulse a few times until almost pasty.

Combine the shrimp in a large bowl with remaining ingredients and mix well to combine.

Using rubber gloves (easier with gloves), form shrimp into 4 patties.

Heat a non-stick skillet over medium heat and spray with oil. Add the shrimp cakes to the heated grill and cook 4 minutes without disturbing, then gently flip and cook an additional 4 minutes.

Serve with fresh lime juice and celeriac mash – see recipe above

133. Sexy Seared Scampi

Ingredients:

2 tsp olive oil

1 1/2 lbs shrimp, peeled and deveined (weight after peeled)

1/4 tsp low sodium salt

1/4 tsp ground black pepper

1/4 tsp crushed red pepper

2 tbsp dry parsley

lemon wedges

Instructions:

Heat 1 tsp oil in 12 inch skillet over high heat until smoking. Meanwhile, toss shrimp with low sodium salt and pepper.

Add half of the shrimp to the pan in single layer and cook until edges turn pink, about 1 minute.

Remove pan from heat, flip shrimp using tongs and let it stand about 30 seconds until all of the shrimp is opaque except for the center.

Transfer to a plate and repeat with the second batch and the remaining teaspoon of oil. After second batch has stood off the heat, add the first batch to the pan and toss to combine.

Cover skillet and let shrimp stand for 1 - 2 minutes. Shrimp will now be cooked through. Serve immediately with a green salad and lemon wedges.

134. Divine Seafood Stew

Ingredients:

3 dozen little clams, scrubbed and clean

1 lb large shrimp, peeled and deveined

1 lb scallops

1 tbsp extra virgin olive oil

4 cloves garlic, minced

1/2 onion, chopped

1 tomato, diced

1 tablespoon dry white wine

1/4 cup water

1 bay leaf

1/2 cup fresh parsley, finely chopped

Low sodium salt and fresh pepper to taste

Instructions:

In a large heavy pot, saute garlic and onion in olive oil over medium flame for about 2 minutes. Add tomatoes, wine, bay leaf, 1/4 cup parsley, low sodium salt and pepper and simmer 5 minutes.

Add the clams, mix well and cover. Cook about 5 minutes or until all the clams open (discard any closed clams).

Add shrimp and scallops and cook an additional 2-3 minutes, until seafood is completely cooked. Ladle into bowls and top with a little fresh parsley.

135. Brussels Mussels

Ingredients:

1 tbsp extra virgin olive oil

1/4 cup minced shallot

1 diced carrot and celery stick

2 garlic cloves, thinly sliced

1 tsp crushed red pepper

1/2 cup dry white wine

3 lbs (48 to 50) live mussels, scrubbed and debearded

2 tbsp chopped parsley, for garnish

Instructions:

In a large saucepan, heat the olive oil over medium-high heat until hot. Add the shallot, garlic and crushed red pepper and cook until fragrant, about 1 minute. Add the wine and boil until reduced by half, about 3 minutes.

Stir in the mussels, cover and cook until the mussels open, 6 to 8 minutes; discard any mussels that do not open. Season lightly with low sodium salt, then transfer the mussels and sauce to a platter. Sprinkle with chopped parsley and serve right away.

136. Roasted Delish Fish Fillet

Ingredients:

3 white fish fillets of choice, 8 oz each

2 tsp olive oil

3 cloves garlic

2 tbsp fresh rosemary or fresh oregano

Low sodium salt and fresh pepper

fresh lemon wedges for serving

Instructions:

Preheat oven to 450°. Rinse and dry fish well. Line a broiler rack with aluminum foil. Lightly spray with oil.

Rub fish with 1 tsp olive oil and season with low sodium salt and pepper, garlic and rosemary.

Place skin side down on oven rack. Drizzle remaining oil and bake until fish is cooked through, about 15-20 minutes.

Serve with cauliflower rice

137. Tantalizing Tuna Steak

Ingredients:

16 oz sushi grade tuna

1 tsp toasted sesame oil

Low sodium salt

fresh pepper

4 cups arugula

For the soy-ginger vinaigrette:

1 tbsp minced ginger

1 tbsp minced green onion

1 tbsp minced garlic

1/2 cup balsamic vinegar

1/4 cup red wine

1/4 cup soy sauce low sodium gluten free

Stevia to taste

2 tsp toasted sesame oil

1 tsp mustard powder

Instructions:

Rub the tuna steaks with 1 tsp oil, and sprinkle with low sodium salt and pepper. Place the tuna steaks in a very hot saute pan and cook for only 1 minute on each side. Set aside on a platter.

Meanwhile, prepare salad and soy vinaigrette. Lightly coat salad with vinaigrette. Slice tuna steaks and place on top of arugula. Drizzle additional vinaigrette over the top.

138. Sexy Creole Prawns

Ingredients:

2 tsp olive oil

1 medium onion, chopped

1/2 cup green bell pepper, chopped

1/2 cup celery, chopped

2 cloves of garlic, minced

14-ounce can of diced tomatoes

8 oz tomato passata

1/4 teaspoon of cayenne pepper

1/4 tsp salt free Cajun Seasoning

1 bay leaf

1 tsp almond flour

2 tbsp water

1 lb of large shrimp, peeled and deveined

1 medium scallion, sliced

2 tbsp fresh parsley, chopped

Low sodium salt to taste

Chilli flakes to taste

Instructions:

In a large skillet heat the olive oil over medium heat. Add the chopped onion, green bell pepper, garlic and celery and saute until tender. Add tomatoes and tomato passata, cayenne pepper, cajun spice, bay leaf and bring to a boil. Cover and reduce heat to low and simmer 20-30 minutes.

Make a slurry of the almond flour and water and stir into the tomato mixture. Continue cooking for another 5 minutes. Lightly season the shrimp with the Cajun seasoning and add immediately to the tomato mixture. Cook for another 5 to 6 minutes, or until shrimp is opaque and cooked through, adjust low sodium salt if needed.

Add chopped green onion and parsley and serve with cauliflower rice.

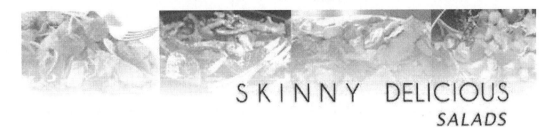

SKINNY DELICIOUS
SALADS

SALAD – ANIMAL PROTEIN

139. Skinny Delicious Slaw
Ingredients:

1/2 head of cabbage   (mix purple and white)

3 or 4 carrots

1 onion

3 tablespoons walnut oil

1 egg beaten

Stevia to taste

1 Tbsp. fresh lemon juice

pepper to taste

Instructions:

Grate cabbage, carrots and onion and mix together.

Make dressing by mixing

beaten egg, walnut oil, lemon juice, and seasonings.

Chill and serve.

140. Turkey Eastern Surprise
Ingredients:

For the salad:

2 cups grilled turkey, chopped

6 baby bok choy, grilled & chopped

2 green onions, chopped

1/4 cup cilantro, chopped

1 Tbl sesame seeds

For the dressing:

1 Tbl fresh ginger, chopped

2 Tbl coconut cream

1 Tbl fish sauce

1 Tbl sesame oil

2 Tbl fresh lime juice

1 tsp stevia powder or to taste

Instructions:

Combine all of the salad ingredients until well mixed.

Add all of the ingredients for the dressing into a blender or food processor, and blend until mostly smooth — there may be some small chunks of ginger left, that's ok.

Pour the dressing over the salad and toss lightly until coated.

Garnish with more sesame seeds if desired.

If possible let it sit for an hour in the fridge before serving so the flavors can really meld together.

141. Mediterranean Turkey Delish Salad
Ingredients:

1 roasted turkey (organic, soy-free and pastured is best)

1/2 cup of olive oil

1/4 cup fresh cilantro, chopped

1 head of romaine or butter lettuce

1 red onion, diced

1 lemon, juiced

low sodium salt and pepper as desired

Instructions:

Shred the turkey with your hands or chop up and put it in a big bowl.

Add the oil, red onion, cilantro, lemon, low sodium salt and pepper.

Mix well and serve on a lettuce boat.

142. Skinny Delicious Turkey Divine
Ingredients:

2/3 cup fresh lime juice

1/3 cup fish sauce

Stevia to taste

3/4 cup chicken stock low sodium

1 1/2 pounds ground turkey

1 cup thinly sliced green onions

3/4 cup thinly sliced shallots

3 tablespoons minced lemongrass

1 tablespoon thinly sliced serrano chile

1/2 cup chopped cilantro leaves

1/3 cup chopped mint leaves

low sodium salt

1 head of any lettuce

Instructions:

Whisk together lime juice, fish sauce, honey and chile-garlic sauce. Set aside.

Warm chicken stock in a medium heavy-bottomed pot over medium heat until simmering. Add ground turkey and simmer until cooked through. As the turkey is cooking, stir occasionally to break up the meat. This should take 6 to 8 minutes.

Add green onion, shallot, lemongrass and chiles, stirring to combine. Continue cooking until shallots turn translucent, stirring occasionally (about 4 minutes). Remove from the heat and drain off any liquid in the pot. I do this by clamping the lid on, then cracking it just a hair. I turn the entire pot over the sink and let the liquid drain out.

Stir in lime juice-fish sauce mixture, cilantro and mint. Season to taste with low sodium salt (not much is needed if any).

Transfer mixture to a large bowl and serve beside a pile of lettuce leaves. Using a slotted spoon, scoop turkey on to the lettuce leaves and enjoy!

143. Chicken Basil Avo Salad

Ingredients:

2 boneless, skinless chicken breasts (organic, cooked and shredded)

1/2 cup fresh basil leaves, stems removed

1 cup sliced cherry tomatoes

2 small or 1 large ripe avocado, pits and skin removed

2 Tbsp. extra virgin olive oil

1/2 tsp. low sodium salt (or more to taste)

1/8 tsp. ground black pepper (or more to taste)

Instructions:

Place the cooked shredded chicken in a medium sized mixing bowl.

Place the basil, avocado, olive oil, low sodium salt and ground black pepper in a food processor and blend until smooth. You may need to scrape the sides a couple times to incorporate.

Pour the avocado and basil mixture into the mixing bowl with the shredded chicken and tomatoes and toss well to coat.

Taste and add additional low sodium salt and ground black pepper if desired. Keep in the fridge until ready to serve.

144. Skinny Chicken salad

Ingredients:

Salad:

1 small head (or 4 cups) savoy cabbage, finely shredded –

1 cup carrot, julienned

1/4 cup scallions, trimmed and julienned

1/4 cup radishes, julienned

1/4 cup fresh cilantro, chopped

1/4 cup fresh mint, chopped

2 cups cooked organic chicken

Vinaigrette:

2 tablespoons coconut or rice vinegar

2 tablespoons sesame oil (use unrefined, expeller or cold-pressed)

juice of 1/2 a lime

1 chipotle pepper (or sub

1 clove garlic, crushed

1 teaspoon fresh ginger, grated

Instructions:

Salad – Combine cabbage, carrots, scallions and radishes. Top with chicken, cilantro and mint and set aside.

Vinaigrette –Combine the vinaigrette ingredients. Taste to see if it needs any adjustments. If it is too spicy, you can add more lime juice to counteract it.

Drizzle salad with vinaigrette & enjoy.

145. Turkey Taco Salad

Ingredients:

1/2 lbs (ish) leftover turkey, cooked and chopped

1 1/2 Tbsp taco seasoning (recipe follows)

1 tsp. coconut or olive oil and 1 tsp rice vinegar

1/4 c. water

Shredded lettuce

Optional Toppings - sliced olives, tomatoes, red onion, avocado, bell peppers,

crushed sweet potato chips

Taco   *Seasoning:*

Mix together, 4 Tbsp. chili powder, 1 tsp each garlic powder, onion powder, and oregano, 2 tsp each paprika and cumin, 4 tsp low sodium salt, and 1/8-1/4 tsp red pepper flakes.

Instructions:

First, make the Raw Ranch Dressing and get that into the fridge to cool.

Then, in a skillet, heat the oil and add in chicken - I like to fry it for a minute to give some extra flavor. Add in water and taco seasoning, let simmer until liquid is gone.

Meanwhile, shred, chop, and dice all your toppings.

Assemble, lettuce, optional toppings, chicken, dressing, and crushed chips.

146. Cheeky Turkey Salad

Ingredients:

For the Turkey:

1 lb boneless turkey breasts

1 tbsp olive oil

low sodium salt and pepper, to taste

For the Salsa:

1 large tomato, quartered

1/2 red onion, cut into large chunks

1 garlic clove, peeled

1 small bunch of cilantro leaves

Juice of 1 lime

low sodium salt and pepper, to taste

Instructions:

Preheat oven to 375 F.

Bake turkey breasts dipped in olive oil on a baking sheet for 35 to 40 minutes, until no longer pink in the center.

While baking, add all salsa ingredients to a food processor and pulse using the chopping blade until finely chopped. Transfer the salsa to a large bowl and clean out the food processor. You will be using it to shred the turkey.

(If you don't have a food processor, just dice the tomato, onion, pepper, cilantro and garlic and add to a bowl with the lime juice, low sodium salt and pepper).

Remove turkey from the oven and allow to cool. Once cool enough to handle, cut each breast into three or four smaller pieces and add to the food processor. Pulse using the chopping blade until shredded.

Add turkey to bowl with salsa and mix well with a fork.

Refrigerate for at least two hours until turkey salad is chilled.

147. Macadamia Chicken Salad
Ingredients:

1lb organic chicken breast

1tsp macadamia nut oil, or oil of choice

few pinches of low sodium salt and pepper

1/2 cup macadamia nuts, chopped

1/2 cup diced celery

2 tbsp julienned basil

1 tablespoon olive oil and 2 teaspoons rice vinegar

1 tbsp lemon juice

Instructions:

Preheat oven to 350. Place chicken breasts on sheet tray, drizzle will oil and a pinch of low sodium salt and pepper. Bake for about 35 minutes until cooked through. Remove from oven and let cool.

In a large bowl shred chicken. Add nuts, celery, basil, dressing, and a pinch of low sodium salt and pepper. Gently stir until combined. Eat!

148. Rosy Chicken Supreme Salad
Ingredients:

For the chicken:

450g chicken mince, free range of course

1 long red chili, finely chopped with the seeds

2 garlic cloves, finely chopped

Little nob of fresh ginger, peeled and finely chopped

1 stem lemon grass, pale section only, finely chopped

1/2 bunch of coriander stems washed and finely chopped (I don't waste anything,

   save the leaves for the salad)

2 1/2 tbsp fish sauce

1/2 lime rind grated

1/2 lime, juiced

A pinch of low sodium salt

Coconut oil for frying (about 3 tablespoons)

For the salad:

1/4 red cabbage, thinly sliced

1 large carrot, peeled and grated

1/2 Spanish onion, thinly sliced

2 tbsp green spring onion, chopped

1/2 bunch of fresh coriander leaves (saved from the stems used in the chicken)

A handful of fresh mint or Thai basil if available

1/2 cup crashed roasted cashews or some sesame seeds

For the dressing:

2 tbsp olive oil

3 tbsp lime juice

1 tbsp fish sauce

1 small red chili, finely chopped

Instructions:

Once you've prepared all your ingredients for the chicken, heat 1 tbsp of coconut oil in a large frying pan or a wok to high.

Throw in lemongrass, chili, garlic, coriander stems and ginger and stir fry for about a minute until fragrant.

Add chicken mince and lime zest. Stir and break apart the mince with a wooden mixing spoon until separated into small chunks (this might take a while as chicken mince is quite sticky).

The meat will now be changing to white colour.

Add fish sauce and lime juice. Stir through and cook for a further few minutes. Total cooking time for the chicken should be about 10 minutes.

Prepare the salad base by mixing together sliced red cabbage, onion grated carrot, and fresh herbs.

Mix all dressing ingredients and toss through the salad.

Serve cooked chicken mince on top of the dressed salad and topped with roasted cashews, dried shallots, coconut flakes and extra fresh herbs.

149. Turkey Sprouts Salad

Ingredients:

1/2 pound of Brussels sprouts (2-ish cups once sliced)

1/2 cup chopped almonds

2 turkey breasts, chopped

1/2 white onion, finely diced

Vinaigrette:

2 TBSP Apple Cider Vinegar

1 TBSP quality mustard powder

1 TBSP avocado oil

Stevia to taste

1/2 tsp low sodium salt

few grinds of black pepper

Instructions:

Cut the Brussels sprouts in half and thinly slice. Chop the half cup of almonds. Finely dice the white onion. Scallions would work too if you prefer a more mild onion flavor... though the white did not overpower.

Remove the breasts and chop into bite-sized pieces. Combine all of these ingredients into a large bowl and gently toss the Brussels sprouts salad.

Whipping up the vinaigrette takes seconds. Add all ingredients to a small bowl and whisk until smooth. Pour over the Brussels sprouts salad and toss to bring together.

150. Delicious Chicken Salad

Ingredients:

Cooked and chopped chicken breast

Chopped almonds

Mashed avocado

Lots of low sodium salt and pepper

Any lettuce leaves of choice

Instructions:

Mix the first six ingredients together in a bowl, season with low sodium salt and pepper, and then spoon onto lettuce leaves. Roll up and enjoy!

151. Avocado Tuna Salad

Ingredients:

2 tins high quality albacore tuna

1 avocado

1/4 of an onion, chopped

juice of 1/2 a lime

2 Tbsp cilantro (or sub basil if you prefer)

some low sodium salt and pepper, to taste

Instructions:

Shred the tuna.

Add all of the other ingredients and mix.

152. Classic Tuna Salad

Ingredients:

2 large grilled tuna steaks

2 tablespoons olive oil

.5 cup onion, chopped (I like red, scallions are also good)

2-3 stalks celery, chopped (or .5 cup)

.5 – .75 cup pecans, chopped (optional)

.5 – 1 tsp low sodium salt

.5 tsp Lemon Garlic pepper

.5 – 1 Tbsp lemon juice

Instructions:

Grill the tuna steaks medium rare with garlic powder and black pepper to taste

Then do a bunch of chopping. Onions, celery, and pecans.

Combine all of these ingredients in the bowl with your cubed tuna and then start adding the dressing of oil and lemon juice seasoned.

You want enough to cover all the ingredients and make them moist, but not overly runny or dry.

It tastes great served right away, but even better after it sits in the fridge for a day.

153. Artichoke Tuna Delight
Ingredients:

1.5 cups diced grilled tuna

¼ cup finely diced red onion

1 small carrot julienned and cut into small pieces (or ½ a diced red bell pepper)

4-5 artichoke hearts (I used canned in water) diced

2 tablespoons capers

low sodium salt and pepper to taste.

6 Radicchio leaves

Instructions:

Place all ingredients, except the radicchio leaves in a large bowl and combine.

Place a scoop if salad into each Radicchio cup and serve.

Store salad in an air tight container in the fridge.

154. Tasty Tuna Stuffed Tomato

Ingredients:

2 large tomatoes

Lettuce leaves (optional)

2 (5 or 6 oz.) cans wild albacore tuna

6 Tbsp. olive oil and 1 tablespoon rice vinegar

1 stalk celery, chopped

1/2 small onion, chopped

1/4 tsp. low sodium salt

1/4 tsp. ground black pepper

Instructions:

Wash and dry the tomatoes and remove any stem. You can either slice off the top part of the tomatoes and hollow them out, or cut each tomato into wedges, making sure to only cut down to about 1/2 inch before you get to the bottom of the tomato.

Arrange the tomatoes on a plate on top of lettuce leaves (optional).

Combine the remaining ingredients in a mixing bowl and add additional low sodium salt and/or pepper if desired. Spoon into the tomatoes and serve.

155. Advanced Avocado Tuna Salad

Ingredients:

1 avocado

1 lemon, juiced, to taste

1 tablespoon chopped onion, to taste

1 cup chopped tomatoes

5 ounces cooked or canned wild tuna

low sodium salt and pepper to taste

Instructions:

Cut the avocado in half and scoop the middle of both avocado halves into a bowl, leaving a shell of avocado flesh about 1/4-inch thick on each half.

Add lemon juice and onion to the avocado in the bowl and mash together.

Add tuna, low sodium salt and pepper, and stir to combine. Taste and adjust if needed.

Fill avocado shells with tuna salad and serve.

156. Sexy Italian Tuna Salad

Ingredients:

10 sun-dried tomatoes

2 (5 oz) can of tuna

1-2 ribs of celery, diced finely

2 Tablespoons of extra virgin olive oil

1 cloves garlic, minced

3 Tablespoons finely chopped parsley

1/2 Tablespoon lemon juice

low sodium salt and pepper to taste

Instructions:

Prepare the sun-dried tomatoes by softening them in warm water for 30 minutes until soft. Then, pat the tomatoes dry and chop finely.

Flake the tuna.

Mix the tuna together with the chopped tomatoes, celery, extra virgin olive oil, garlic, parsley, and lemon juice. Add low sodium salt and pepper to taste.

If not serving immediately, mix with extra olive oil just before serving.

Optional: Make cucumber boats with them.

157. Divine Chicken or Turkey and Baby Bok Choy Salad

Ingredients:

For the salad:

2 cups grilled chicken or turkey, chopped

6 baby bok choy, grilled & chopped

2 green onions, chopped

1/4 cup cilantro, chopped

1 Tbsp sesame seeds

For the dressing:

1 Tbsp fresh ginger, chopped

2 Tbsp coconut cream

1 Tbsp soy sauce

1 Tbsp sesame oil

2 Tbsp fresh lime juice

1 Tsp stevia powder

Instructions:

Combine all of the salad ingredients until well mixed.

Add all of the ingredients for the dressing into a blender or food processor, and blend until mostly smooth

Pour the dressing over the salad and toss lightly until coated.

Garnish with more sesame seeds if desired.

158. Mediterranean Medley Salad

Ingredients:

1 roasted chicken (organic, soy-free and pastured is best).. or turkey or ostrich steak

Dressing:

1/2 cup of olive oil, ¼ cup apple cider vinegar and garlic powder and chilli powder to taste

1/4 cup fresh cilantro, chopped

1 head of romaine or butter lettuce

1 red onion, diced

1 lemon, juiced

low sodium salt and pepper as desired

Instructions:

Shred the chicken/turkey etc or chop up and put it in a big bowl.

Add the dressing…also red onion, cilantro, lemon, low sodium salt and pepper.

Mix well and serve on a lettuce boat.

159. Spicy Eastern Salad

Ingredients:

2/3 cup fresh lime juice

1/3 cup fish sauce(optional)

Stevia to taste

3/4 cup low sodium chicken stock (preferably homemade)

1 1/2 pounds ground chicken or turkey

1 cup thinly sliced green onions

3/4 cup thinly sliced shallots

3 tablespoons minced lemongrass

1 tablespoon thinly sliced serrano chilli

1/2 cup chopped cilantro leaves

1/3 cup chopped mint leaves

Low sodium salt

1 head of butter lettuce or other green leaves

Instructions:

Whisk together lime juice, fish sauce (optional – try low sodium version)..stevia and Set aside.

Warm chicken stock in a medium heavy-bottomed pot over medium heat until simmering.

Add ground chicken and simmer until cooked through. As the chicken is cooking, stir occasionally to break up the meat. This should take 6 to 8 minutes.

Add green onion, shallot, lemongrass and chilies, stirring to combine. Continue cooking until shallots turn translucent, stirring occasionally (about 4 minutes).

Remove from the heat and drain off any liquid in the pot. I do this by clamping the lid on, then cracking it just a hair. I turn the entire pot over the sink and let the liquid drain out.

Stir in lime juice-fish sauce mixture, cilantro and mint. Season to taste with low sodium salt (not much is needed if any).

Transfer mixture to a large bowl and serve beside a pile of lettuce leaves. Using a slotted spoon, scoop on to the lettuce leaves and enjoy!

160. Basil Avocado Bonanza Salad

Ingredients:

2 boneless, skinless chicken or turkey breasts (cooked and shredded)

1/2 cup fresh basil leaves, stems removed

2 small or 1 large ripe avocado, pits and skin removed

2 Tbsp. extra virgin olive oil

1/2 tsp. low sodium salt (or more to taste)

1/8 tsp. ground black pepper (or more to taste)

Instructions:

Place the cooked shredded chicken in a medium sized mixing bowl.

Place the basil, avocado, olive oil, low sodium salt and ground black pepper in a food processor and blend until smooth.

Pour the avocado and basil mixture into the mixing bowl with the shredded chicken and toss well to coat.

Taste and add additional low sodium salt and ground black pepper if desired. Keep in the fridge until ready to serve.

161. Chinese Divine Salad

Ingredients:

Salad :

1 small head (or 4 cups) savoy cabbage, finely shredded –

1 cup carrot, julienned (about 1 large carrot)

1/4 cup scallions, trimmed and julienned (about 3 scallions)

1/4 cup radishes, julienned

1/4 cup fresh cilantro, chopped

1/4 cup fresh mint, chopped

2 cups cooked chicken or turkey

*Vinaigrette***:**

2 tablespoons coconut or rice vinegar

Low sodium salt to taste

2 tablespoons sesame oil

1 chipotle pepper

1/2 teaspoon chilli flakes

1 clove garlic, crushed

1 teaspoon fresh ginger, grated

Stevia to taste

Instructions:

Salad – Combine cabbage, carrots, scallions and radishes. Top with chicken, cilantro and mint and set aside.

Vinaigrette –Combine the vinaigrette ingredients. Taste to see if it needs any adjustments. If it is too spicy, you can add more lime juice to counteract it.

Drizzle salad with vinaigrette & enjoy

162. Divinely Delish Salad Surprise
Ingredients:

1/2 lbs leftover chicken, turkey or boiled egg cooked and chopped

1 tsp. coconut or olive oil

1/4 c. water

Shredded lettuce

Optional Toppings - sliced olives, tomatoes, red onion, avocado, bell peppers

Non-optional Toppings - crushed sweet potato chips

Divine Dressing:

Mix together, 4 Tbsp. chili powder, 1 tsp each garlic powder, onion powder, and oregano, 2 tsp each paprika and cumin, 4 tsp low sodium salt, and 1/8-1/4 tsp red pepper flakes. Add 1 cup olive oil and half cup rice vinegar

Instructions:

Then, in a skillet, heat the oil and add in chicken etc –. Add in water let simmer until liquid is gone.

Meanwhile, shred, chop, and dice all your toppings.

Assemble, lettuce, optional toppings, chicken, dressing, and crushed chips.

Add Divine Dressing.

163. Avocado Salad with Cilantro and Lime
Ingredients:

Turkey Breast chopped

Two avocados, diced

2/3 green cabbage, chopped

5 green onions (scallions), white and pale green parts, minced

Juice of 2 limes

Two handfuls of fresh cilantro, chopped

low sodium salt to taste

One large English Cucumber

Instructions:

Mix all ingredients except cucumber -slice it thinly and use it as a base for the salad. For "party style", slice 1-2 inch sections, scoop out the center with a grapefruit spoon, and fill the cucumber "cups" with the salad.

Divine Dressing:

Mix together, 4 Tbsp. chili powder, 1 tsp each garlic powder, onion powder, and oregano, 2 tsp each paprika and cumin, 4 tsp low sodium salt, and 1/8-1/4 tsp red pepper flakes. Add 1 cup olive oil and half cup rice vinegar.

164. Mexican Medley Salad

Ingredients:

For the Chicken or turkey:

1 lb boneless chicken/turkey breasts

1 tbsp olive oil

low sodium salt and pepper, to taste

For the Salsa:

1 large tomato, quartered

1/2 red onion, cut into large chunks

1 jalapeno pepper, stem and seeds removed and halved

1 garlic clove, peeled

1 small bunch of cilantro leaves

Juice of 1 lime

low sodium salt and pepper, to taste

Instructions:

Preheat oven to 375 F.

Brush chicken breasts on both sides with olive oil and sprinkle with low sodium salt and pepper. Bake on a baking sheet for 35 to 40 minutes, until no longer pink in the center.

While chicken is baking, add all salsa ingredients to a food processor and pulse using the chopping blade until finely chopped.

Transfer the salsa to a large bowl and clean out the food processor. You will be using it to shred the chicken.

Remove chicken from the oven and allow to cool. Once cool enough to handle, cut each breast into three or four smaller pieces and add to the food processor. Pulse using the chopping blade until shredded.

Add chicken to bowl with salsa and mix well with a fork.

Refrigerate for at least two hours until chicken salad is chilled.

165. Macadamia Nut Chicken/Turkey Salad
Ingredients:

1lb chicken/turkey breast

1tsp macadamia nut oil, or oil of choice

few pinches of low sodium salt and pepper

1/2 cup macadamia nuts, chopped

1/2 cup diced celery

3 tbsp divine dressing

2 tbsp julienned basil

1 tbsp lemon juice

Instructions:

Preheat oven to 350. Place chicken breasts on sheet tray, drizzle will oil and a pinch of low sodium salt and pepper.

Bake for about 35 minutes until cooked through. Remove from oven and let cool.

In a large bowl shred chicken. Add nuts, celery, basil, mayo, lemon juice, and a pinch of low sodium salt and pepper. Gently stir until combined. Eat!

Divine Dressing:

Mix together, 4 Tbsp. chili powder, 1 tsp each garlic powder, onion powder, and oregano, 2 tsp each paprika and cumin, 4 tsp low sodium salt, and 1/8-1/4 tsp red pepper flakes. Add 1 cup olive oil and half cup rice vinegar.

166. Red Cabbage Bonanza Salad

Ingredients:

For the chicken or turkey:

450g chicken/turkey mince, free range of course

1 long red chili, finely chopped with the seeds

2 garlic cloves, finely chopped

Little nob of fresh ginger, peeled and finely chopped

1 stem lemon grass, pale section only, finely chopped

1/2 bunch of coriander stems washed and finely chopped (I don't waste anything, save the leaves for the salad)

1 tbsp low sodium salt

1 tbsp coconut aminos

1/2 lime rind grated

1/2 lime, juiced

A pinch of low sodium salt

Coconut oil for frying (about 3 tablespoons)

For the salad:

1/4 red cabbage, thinly sliced

1 large carrot, peeled and grated

1/2 Spanish onion, thinly sliced

2 tbsps green spring onion, chopped

1/2 bunch of fresh coriander leaves (saved from the stems used in the chicken)

A handful of fresh mint or Thai basil if available

1/2 cup crashed roasted cashews or some sesame seeds

1/2 cup dried fried shallots (optional for garnish)

2 tbsp toasted coconut flakes (optional for garnish)

For the dressing:

2 tbsp olive oil

3 tbsps lime juice

1 small red chili, finely chopped (you can leave it out if you like it mild)

Instructions:

Once you've prepared all your ingredients for the chicken, heat 1 tbsp of coconut oil in a large frying pan or a wok to high. Throw in lemongrass, chili, garlic, coriander stems and ginger and stir fry for about a minute until fragrant.

Add chicken mince and lime zest. Stir and break apart the mince with a wooden mixing spoon until separated into small

The meat will now be changing to white colour. Add lime juice. Stir through and cook for a further few minutes. Total cooking time for the chicken should be about 10 minutes.

Prepare the salad base by mixing together sliced red cabbage, onion grated carrot, and fresh herbs.

Mix all dressing ingredients and toss through the salad.

Serve cooked chicken mince on top of the dressed salad and topped with roasted cashews, dried shallots, coconut flakes and extra fresh herbs.

167. Spectacular Sprouts Salad

Ingredients:

1/2 pound of mixed sprouts (2-ish cups once sliced)

1/2 Granny Smith apple

1/2 cup chopped almonds

2 chicken breasts, chopped

1/2 white onion, finely diced

Vinaigrette:

2 TBSP Apple Cider Vinegar

1 TBSP quality brown mustard

1 TBSP avocado oil

Stevia to taste

1/2 tsp low sodium salt

few grinds of black pepper

Instructions:

Cut Granny Smith apple, slicing into matchsticks.

Chop the half cup of almonds. Finely dice the white onion. Scallions would work too if you prefer a more mild onion flavor... though the white did not overpower.

Remove the breasts and chop into bite-sized pieces. Combine all of these ingredients into a large bowl and gently toss the sprouts into the salad.

Whipping up the vinaigrette takes seconds. Add all ingredients to a small bowl and whisk until smooth. Pour over the sprouts salad and toss to bring together.

168. Avocado Egg Salad

Ingredients:

Cooked and chopped organic eggs x 3

Chopped almonds

Mashed avocado

low sodium salt and pepper

Any lettuce leaves

Instructions:

Mix the ingredients together in a bowl, season with low sodium salt and pepper, and then spoon onto lettuce leaves. Roll up and enjoy!

169. Avocado Divine Salad

Ingredients:

1 kilo boneless, skinless chicken or turkey breasts (2 or 3)

1 avocado

1/4 of an onion, chopped

juice of one lime and one lemon

2 tbsps cilantro (or sub basil if you prefer)

some low sodium salt and pepper, to taste

One bag mixed lettuce leaves

One tablespoon olive oil

Instructions:

Cook chicken breast until done, let cool, and then shred. Add all of the other ingredients and mix.

170. Classic Waldorf Salad

Ingredients:

half whole cooked chicken or turkey (~2lbs)

half cup apple, peeled and chopped (optional)

half cup onion, chopped (I like red, scallions are also good)

2-3 stalks celery, chopped (or .5 cup)

half cup pecans, chopped (optional)

half tsp low sodium salt

half tsp Lemon Garlic

pepper

1 tbsp lemon juice

Divine Dressing:

Mix together, 4 Tbsp. chili powder, 1 tsp each garlic powder, onion powder, and oregano, 2 tsp each paprika and cumin, 4 tsp low sodium salt, and 1/8-1/4 tsp red pepper flakes. Add 1 cup olive oil and half cup rice vinegar

Instructions:

First cook up a whole chicken. You can buy a rotisserie chicken, or do what I do, throw a chicken in the crockpot, sprinkle it with cumin, low sodium salt & pepper and let it cook for about 4-6 hours on low.

After the chicken is cooked and cooled, de-bone and shred the meat (white and dark) and put it in a large mixing bowl. I usually use about half of my 3-4lb chicken.

Then do a bunch of chopping. Peel your apple, then chop your apple, onions, celery, and pecans.

Combine all of these ingredients in the bowl with your chicken and then start adding the dressing. You want enough to cover all the ingredients and make them moist, but not overly runny or dry.

Add the low sodium salt and pepper, and lemon juice Stir well to combine. Add dressing.

171. Artichoke Heart & Turkey Salad Radicchio Cups

Ingredients:

1.5 cups diced cooked turkey

¼ cup finely diced red onion

1 small carrot julienned and cut into small pieces (or ½ a diced red bell pepper)

4-5 artichoke hearts (I used canned in water) diced low sodium salt and pepper to taste.

6 Radicchio leaves

Instructions:

Place all ingredients, except the radicchio leaves in a large bowl and combine.

Place a scoop if salad into each Radicchio cup and serve.

Store salad in an air tight container in the fridge.

Divine Dressing:

Mix together, 4 Tbsp. chili powder, 1 tsp each garlic powder, onion powder, and oregano, 2 tsp each paprika and cumin, 4 tsp low sodium salt, and 1/8-1/4 tsp red pepper flakes. Add 1 cup olive oil and half cup rice vinegar.

172. Tempting Tuna Stuffed Tomato
Ingredients:

2 large tomatoes

Lettuce leaves (optional)

2 (5 or 6 oz.) cans wild albacore tuna

1 stalk celery, chopped

1/2 small onion, chopped

1/4 tsp. low sodium salt

1/4 tsp. ground black pepper

Instructions:

Wash and dry the tomatoes and remove any stem.

Arrange the tomatoes on a plate on top of lettuce leaves (optional).

Combine the remaining ingredients in a mixing bowl and add additional low sodium salt and/or pepper if desired.

Spoon into the tomatoes and serve.

173. Incredibly Delish Avocado Tuna Salad

Ingredients:

1 avocado

1 lemon, juiced, to taste

1 tablespoon chopped onion, to taste

5 ounces cooked or canned wild tuna

low sodium salt and pepper to taste

Instructions:

Cut the avocado in half and scoop the middle of both avocado halves into a bowl, leaving a shell of avocado flesh about 1/4-inch thick on each half.

Add lemon juice and onion to the avocado in the bowl and mash together. Add tuna, low sodium salt and pepper, and stir to combine. Taste and adjust if needed.

Fill avocado shells with tuna salad and serve.

174. Italian Tuna Bonanza Salad

Ingredients:

10 sun-dried tomatoes

2 (5 oz) can of tuna

1-2 ribs of celery, diced finely

2 Tablespoons of extra virgin olive oil

1 cloves garlic, minced

3 Tablespoons finely chopped parsley

1/2 Tablespoon lemon juice

low sodium salt and pepper to taste

Instructions:

Prepare the sun-dried tomatoes by softening them in warm water for 30 minutes until soft. Then, pat the tomatoes dry and chop finely.

Flake the tuna. and mix the tuna together with the chopped tomatoes, celery, extra virgin olive oil, garlic, parsley, and lemon juice. Add low sodium salt and pepper to taste.

If not serving immediately, mix with extra olive oil just before serving.

Optional: Make cucumber boats with them.

175. Asian Aspiration Salad
Ingredients:

1 red bell pepper, sliced

1 large carrot, cut into matchsticks

1 cucumber, halved lengthwise and sliced

Optional:

fresh ginger juice and rice vinegar

2 boiled eggs

Instructions:

Mix ingredients and Serve.

176. Tasty Carrot Salad
Ingredients:

5 carrots, medium

1 tbs. whole black mustard seeds

1/4 tsp. low sodium salt

2 tsp. lemon juice

2 tbs. olive oil

Add 1 Grated egg on top

Instructions:

Trim and peel and grate carrots. In a bowl, toss with low sodium salt and set aside.

In a small heavy pan over medium heat, heat oil.

When very hot, add mustard seeds. As soon as the seeds begin to pop, in a few seconds, pour oil and seeds over carrots.

Add lemon juice and toss. Serve at room temperature or cold.

Add Grated egg.

177. Creamy Carrot Salad
Ingredients:

1 pound carrots - shredded

20 ounces crushed pineapple -- drained

8 ounces Coconut milk

3/4 cup flaked coconut

Stevia to taste

Shredded turkey one breast

Instructions:

Combine all ingredients, tossing well. Cover and chill.

178. Sublime Courgette Tomato Salad
Ingredients:

2 medium zucchini

2 tomatoes

cooking spray

low sodium salt

freshly ground black pepper

a few sprigs fresh parsley

Instructions:

Heat your grill to high flame.

Wash zucchini and trim off the ends. Using a mandolin or vegetable peeler slice the zucchini lengthwise in thin slices.

Lightly spray with cooking spray and season with low sodium salt and pepper, to taste. Grill the zucchini ribbons on 1 side, until lightly marked and wilted, about 1 to 2 minutes. Remove and put on a platter and let cool slightly.

Cut up tomatoes in large chunks, season with low sodium salt and pepper to taste. Arrange on a platter with zucchini and garnish with parsley sprigs.

179. Brussels Muscles Sprouts
Ingredients:

6 oz brussels sprouts, washed

2 tbsp olive oil

juice of 1 large lemon

low sodium salt and fresh cracked pepper, to taste

Instructions:

With a large sharp knife, trim off the stems, cut the brussels in half lengthwise, then place cut side down on the board and finely shred the sprouts.

Place in a large bowl and toss with olive oil, lemon juice, low sodium salt and pepper to taste.

180. Blushing Beet Salad
Ingredients:

2 large beets, washed and stems cut off

1 cup carrots, peeled and cooked

1 tbsp cilantro, chopped

1 tbsp diced onion

2 tbsp paleo mayonnaise

Low sodium salt and pepper

Instructions:

Boil beets in water until soft, about 50 minutes. Peel and cut into small 1/2" cubes. Cook carrots until tender and cut into bite size cubes. Combine diced onion, carrots, beets, mayonnaise, cilantro, low sodium salt and pepper.

181. Sashimi Divine with Vinaigrette
Ingredients:

5 oz sashimi tuna (sushi grade)

1 tsp extra virgin olive oil

1 tsp fresh lemon juice

2 cups baby arugula

1 tsp capers

Low sodium salt and fresh pepper

Instructions:

Season tuna with low sodium salt and fresh cracked pepper.

Place arugula and capers on a plate. Combine oil and lemon juice, low sodium salt and pepper.

Heat your grill to high heat and clean grate well. When grill is hot, spray grate with oil to prevent sticking then place tuna on the grill; cook one minute without moving. Turnover and cook an additional minute; remove from heat and set aside on a plate.

Slice tuna on the diagonal and place on top of salad. Top with lemon vinaigrette and eat immediately.

182. Grilled Shrimp Fennel Salad
Ingredients:

1 lb jumbo shrimp, peeled and deveined (weight after peeled)

4 cups fresh arugula or baby greens

1 cup (1/2 small bulb) fresh fennel, thinly sliced or shaved w/ mandoline

1 medium-size ripe Hass avocado, sliced thin

For the vinaigrette:

3 tbsp fresh lemon juice

1 tbsp extra-virgin olive oil

3 tbsp minced shallots

 Low sodium salt, to taste

freshly ground black pepper, to taste

Instructions:

For the vinaigrette:

Combine the lemon juice, olive oil, shallots, low sodium salt and pepper in a container with a tight-fitting lid and shake it vigorously to combine.

Reserve 1⁄2 cup of the vinaigrette for dressing the salad and pour the remaining vinaigrette into a medium nonreactive bowl. Put the shrimp in the bowl, season with low sodium salt and pepper and toss; let it sit for about 30 minutes.

Prepare your outdoor grill, or heat a grill pan over medium-high heat. Grill the shrimp until just cooked through and opaque, about 1 1/2 minutes per side. Transfer to a plate.

Divide the baby greens on four plates, top with sliced fennel, oranges, avocados and shrimp. Season with low sodium salt and pepper to taste and drizzle with the remaining vinaigrette, about 2 tbsp per salad.

183. Chicken Delish Salad

Ingredients:

1 lb skinless boneless chicken breast, cut into 1 inch cubes

For the marinade:
2 tbsp fresh squeezed lemon juice

1 tsp dried oregano

1 tsp garlic, crushed

Low sodium salt to taste

fresh ground black pepper to taste

For the salad:

1 1/4 cups cucumber, peeled

1 1/4 cups diced tomato

1/4 cup diced bell pepper

2 tbsp red onion, diced

1 1/2 tsp vinegar

1 1/2 tsp fresh lemon juice

2 tsp olive oil

1 tsp fresh parsley

1/8 tsp dried oregano

Low sodium salt and black pepper to taste

4 cups shredded lettuce

lemon wedges for serving

Instructions:

Marinate the chicken at least 2-3 hours or overnight. If using wooden skewers, soak in water at least 30 minutes if grilling outdoors.

Combine the first 12 salad ingredients (cucumbers through low sodium salt and black pepper, not the lettuce) and set aside in the refrigerator to let the flavors set.

Thread chicken on 4 skewers and cook on a hot grill (indoor or outdoor grill) until chicken is cooked though, about 10-12 minutes.

Divide lettuce between four plates, top with tomato-cucumber salad, and grilled chicken. Serve with lemon wedges.

184. Sea Scallops Sensation

Ingredients:

For the dressing:

1 tbsp red wine vinegar

1 tbsp cider vinegar

2 tbsp olive oil

1 tsp minced shallots

4 drops tbsp stevia

For the salad:

2 cups diced cooked and peeled beets

12 large sea scallops (18 oz)

olive oil cooking spray

low sodium salt and pepper to taste

5 oz baby arugula

8 grape tomatoes, halved

Instructions:

Cover the beets with water in a medium pot and bring to a boil. Cover and cook over medium-low heat until tender when pierced with a fork, about 50 to 60 minutes. Peel and dice into small cubes; set aside to cool.

Season scallops with low sodium salt and pepper. Heat a large nonstick pan on a medium-high heat. When the pan is hot, spray with oil and place scallops in the pan. Sear without touching them until the bottom forms a nice caramel colored crust, about 2 to 3 minutes. Turn and cook until their centers are still slightly translucent (you can check this by viewing them from the side), about 1 to 2 more minutes, careful not to overcook. Remove from the pan.

Make vinaigrette by whisking the dressing ingredients in a small bowl. Toss with the arugula. Evenly divide the arugula between four large plates. Top each with 1/2 cup beet, tomato and 3 scallops each. Serve immediately.

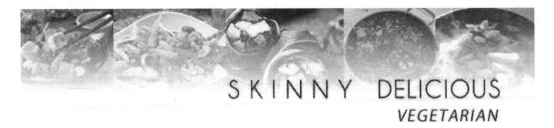

SKINNY DELICIOUS
VEGETARIAN

PURE VEGETABLES

185. Vegetarian Curry with Squash

Ingredients:

1 tbsp coconut oil

2 cups mixed raw nuts.

1 medium yellow onion, diced

1 tsp low sodium salt

1 green bell pepper, thinly sliced

4 cloves garlic, minced

1-inch piece fresh ginger, peeled and minced

1 14-oz. can coconut milk

1 large acorn squash, peeled, seeded, and cut into 1-inch cubes

2 tsp lime juice

One teaspoon curry powder (mild or hot)

1/4 cup cilantro, chopped

Cauliflower rice, for serving

Instructions:

Melt the coconut oil in a large pan over medium heat. Add the onion and cook for 5-6 minutes, stirring occasionally. Add the bell pepper, garlic, ginger, and low sodium salt and stir to combine. Cook for an additional minute.

Add the curry powder to the pan and cook for about a minute, stirring to coat the other ingredients. Add in the coconut milk and bring to a simmer. Stir in the squash.

Simmer, stirring occasionally, for 15-20 minutes until the squash is fork-tender. Remove the pan from the heat and stir in the lime juice. Taste and adjust low sodium salt and lime juice as necessary. Sprinkle with cilantro to serve.

Roast the nuts under the grill until crisp and sprinkle over the top of the curry.

186. Saucy Gratin with Creamy Cauliflower Bonanza

Ingredients:

1 medium butternut squash, peeled, seeded, and diced

1 large sweet potato, peeled and thinly sliced

6 cups fresh spinach

1 tbsp extra virgin olive oil

2 large shallots, diced

4 cloves garlic, chopped

low sodium salt and pepper, to taste

Pinch of nutmeg

For the sauce:

1/2 head of cauliflower, cut into florets

1 cup almond milk

1/2 cup low sodium chicken stock

1/2 tsp low sodium salt

1/2 tsp freshly ground pepper

1/4 tsp nutmeg

Instructions:

Preheat the oven to 375 degrees F. To make the cream sauce, place a couple inches of water in a large pot. Once the water is boiling, place steamer insert and then cauliflower florets into the pot and cover. Steam for 12-14 minutes, until completely tender.

Drain and return cauliflower to the pot. Add the almond milk, stock, nutmeg, low sodium salt, and pepper to the pot. Use an immersion blender or food processor to combine the ingredients until smooth. Set aside.

Meanwhile, bring a separate pot of water to a boil. Add the butternut squash and cook for 4 minutes. Drain and set aside.

Heat the oil in a small pan over medium heat. Add the shallots and garlic and cook for 4-5 minutes until soft. Stir in the spinach to wilt. Season with low sodium salt and pepper.

To assemble, grease a large baking dish with coconut oil spray. Spoon a thin layer of the cream sauce over the bottom of the pan.

Arrange a layer of half of the butternut squash. Top with half of the spinach mixture, and then all of the sliced sweet potato.

Drizzle with the cream sauce. Add the remaining half of the spinach, followed by the rest of the butternut squash. Drizzle the rest of the cream sauce over the top.

Sprinkle with low sodium salt, pepper, and nutmeg. Bake for 50-60 minutes until browned. Allow to cool for 10 minutes.

187. Egg Bok Choy and Basil Stir-Fry

Ingredients:

1 tablespoon fish sauce (I used Red Boat)

1 garlic clove, minced

3 organic eggs

2 tablespoons olive oil

1 small onion, finely chopped

1-inch piece fresh ginger, chopped

2 red chiles, thinly sliced crosswise

1 cup thinly sliced bok choy stems

1 cup thinly sliced bok choy greens

handful fresh basil leaves, chopped

juice of 1 lime

Instructions:

In a large bowl mix fish sauce, garlic and ginger.

Heat the olive oil in a wok (or a large nonstick skillet) over medium-high heat.

Once it starts to shimmer add onion and chiles. Stir-fry the onions until they start to brown around the edges, about 2 minutes.

Stir in the bok choy stems and stir-fry for 1 minute.

Add the beaten eggs and cook until it's nearly cooked through about 2 minutes, stirring often.

Stir in bok choy greens, basil and lime juice. And stir-fry for 30 seconds or so, until the greens are wilted. Serve immediately.

188. Skinny Eggie Vegetable Stir Fry
Ingredients:

1 lb of Cubed Butternut Squash

1 lb of Green Beans

3 Baby Bok Choys

1½ lb of Eggplants

3 Garlic Cloves

1 small Yellow Onion

½ teaspoon of low sodium salt

½ teaspoon of Black Pepper

1-2 Tablespoons of coconut oil

3 organic eggs

Instructions:

Peel, core, and cut the butternut squash into 1" cubes.

Snap the ends off the green beans and slice at an angle into 1.5" long pieces.

Chop the bok choy leaves from the stems. Slice the stems into 1" thick pieces. Cut the leaves in half.

Slice the eggplants into 1" thick discs, then quarter the disc into wedges. Slice in half if the eggplant is skinny.

Mince the garlic cloves and slice the onions.

Heat a wok and add the cooking oil.

Add the onions and cook until translucent. About 2 minutes.

Add the garlic and cook for another minute.

Add the squash, beans (see note), low sodium salt, pepper

Add the eggplant and bok choy stalks and cook uncovered for another 7-10 minutes.

Add the bok choy leaves and cook for another few minutes, covered.

Beat the eggs and add them to the stir fry ...keep stirring till they are cooked through

189. Rucola Salad

Ingredients:

4 teaspoons fresh lemon juice

4 teaspoons walnut oil

low sodium salt and freshly ground pepper

6 cups rucola leaves and tender stems (about 6 ounces)

Garlic powder to taste

Instructions:

Pour the lemon juice into a large bowl. Gradually whisk in the oil. Season with low sodium salt and pepper.

Add the greens, toss until evenly dressed and serve at once. This is delicious, and feel free to add tomatoes or grated carrot and onion slices.

Substitution: Any mild green, such as lamb's lettuce will do.

190. Tasty Spring Salad

Ingredients:

5 cups of any salad greens in season of your choice

Dressing:

125 mL (1/2 cup) olive oil

45 mL (3 tbsp) lemon juice

15 mL (1 tbsp) pure mustard powder

45 mL (3 tbsp) capers, minced (optional)

low sodium salt

pepper

Instructions:

Combine salad greens and any other raw vegetables of choice.

Combine oil, lemon juice and mustard. Mix well.

Add capers, low sodium salt and pepper to taste.

Pour dressing over salad, toss and serve.

191. Spinach and Dandelion Pomegranate Salad

Ingredients:

1 small bunch fresh spinach

12 dandelion leaves

1 cup pomegranate seeds

1/2 cup pecan halves

Instructions:

You may substitute appropriate fresh greens for the dandelion and sorrel leaves.

Wash and destem spinach. Pick and wash sorrel and dandelions.

Coarsely chop dandelion leaves, and tear spinach, then toss dandelion, sorrel and spinach together in a stainless steel bowl.

Put aside in refrigerator to drain and cool.

When drained, pour off excess water, and add pomegranate and pecans. Toss with dressing and serve.

192. Pure Delish Spinach Salad

Ingredients:

2 bunches fresh spinach

1 bunch scallions, chopped

juice of 1 lemon

1/4 tbsp olive oil

pepper to taste

optional: rice vinegar to taste

Instructions:

Wash spinach well. Drain and chop.

After a few minutes, squeeze excess water.

Add scallions, lemon juice, oil and pepper.

193. Sexy Salsa Salad

Ingredients:

1 bunch of cilantro

5-6 roma tomatoes

1 small yellow or red onion

1 small chili pepper

2 ripe avocados.

handful of rucola leaf

Instructions:

Chop cilantro, dice tomatoes, dice onion, finely dice chili pepper, dice avocado.

After dicing each ingredient add to large bowl. Add rucola to bowl.

When finished, toss.

194. Eastern Avo Salad

Ingredients:

2 to 3 lbs. of tomatoes

4 med. or lg. avocados (or 1lb chopped or ground nuts or seeds)

4 stalks celery

4 lg. red (or green) bell peppers

2 lbs. bok choy stalks and greens

Instructions:

Dice the tomatoes, celery and the bell peppers.

Quarter, peel and dice the avocados.

Cut up the bok choy.

Place all ingredients in a bowl and mix together.

195. Curry Coconut Salad

Ingredients:

6 large ripe tomatoes, peeled, seeded and chopped

1 small white onion, grated

1/4 tsp. coarsely ground pepper

1/2 cup coconut cream

2 Tbsp minced fresh parsley

1 tsp. curry powder

Instructions:

Combine tomatoes, onion and pepper; cover and chill for 3 hours.

Combine coconut cream, parsley and curry; cover and chill for 3 hours.

To serve, spoon tomato mixture into small bowls and top each with a spoonful of coconut cream mixture.

196. Jalapeno Salsa
Ingredients:

1 jalapeno pepper seeded and chopped fine

2 large ripe tomatoes, peeled and chopped

1 medium onion, minced

2 tbsp olive oil

juice of 1 lemon

1/2 tsp dried oregano

pepper to taste

Instructions:

Combine all ingredients and mix well. Refrigerate covered until ready to eat.

197. Beet Sprout Divine Salad
Ingredients:

1/2 pound Brussels sprouts, ends trimmed, outer leaves removed, and cut in half lengthwise

4 small red beets, tops trimmed to 1/2-inch, washed and cut in half lengthwise

4 tablespoons plus 1/3 cup extra virgin olive oil

1 tablespoon paleo Dijon mustard

Stevia to taste

Squeeze of lemon juice

Coarse low sodium salt

Grinding coarse black pepper

1 small red onion thinly sliced into rings

Instructions:

Preheat the oven to 350.

Pour 2 tablespoons olive oil in a baking dish. Toss the Brussels sprouts in the oil; sprinkle them with low sodium salt and pepper and roast them for 20 minutes.

Turn them once during the cooking. They are done when a small knife easily pierces them.

Pour 2 tablespoons of the olive oil on a sheet of aluminum foil and place

it on a baking sheet. Toss the beet halves in the olive oil. Sprinkle them with low sodium salt and pepper and, keeping them in a single layer, fold and seal the foil over them. Bake on the baking sheet until a knife easily pierces them.

When cool enough to handle, peel the beets and cut them into 1/4-inch slices.

Meanwhile combine the 1/3 cup olive oil, mustard, stevia, lemon juice and low sodium salt and pepper in a small bowl.

Toss the Ingredients, add the dressing and serve at room temperature.

198. Divine Carrot Salad

Ingredients:

3 tablespoons fresh lemon juice

1 tablespoon Olive oil

1 pressed garlic clove

1-1/2 pound carrots, peeled and rectangle and lightly steamed

Instructions:

Mix dressing ingredients in a small bowl. Add carrots; toss to mix.

Let stand at room temperature for one hour and then serve.

199. Cauliflower Couscous

Ingredients:

1 1/2 Lbs cauliflower florets

1/2 cup parsley (VERY finely chopped)

1/2 cup fresh mint (very FINELY chopped)

1/2 cup chopped red onion

One cucumber finely cubed

4.5 to 5 Tbls fresh lime juice (about 2 fruits)

2 Tbls olive oil

1 teas low sodium salt

1 teas black pepper

Instructions:

In a food processor (NOT A BLENDER) pulse cauliflower until it looks like

rice. Set aside in serving bowl

In food processor- blend parsley, mint, onion, lime juice, olive oil, and low sodium salt and pepper into a smooth paste.

Pour over cauliflower and cucumber and blend well.

200. Mouthwatering Mushroom Salad

Ingredients:

2/3 cup olive oil

1/3 cup fresh lemon juice

One tablespoon red wine vinegar

1 tsp dried thyme

pepper and garlic powder to taste

1 pound fresh mushrooms, thinly sliced

1/4 cup minced parsley

Rucola leaves

Instructions:

Combine all ingredients except the mushrooms, parsley and greens, and mix well.

Add the mushrooms and toss with 2 forks. Cover and let stand at room temperature.

At serving time, drain and sprinkle with the parsley. Pile in a serving dish lined with greens.

201. Skinny Sweet Potato Salad

Ingredients:

4 small sweet potatoes

1 tablespoon olive oil extra virgin

1 teaspoon mustard powder

4 celery stalks, sliced 1/4-inch thick

1 small red bell pepper, cut into 1/4-inch dice

2 scallions, finely chopped

low sodium salt and pepper

1/2 cup coarsely chopped toasted pecans

Chopped fresh chives

Instructions:

Preheat oven to 400°F.

Wrap each sweet potato in foil and bake for 1 hour.

Unwrap; let cool. Peel; cut into 3/4-inch chunks.

In a large bowl, mix oil and mustard. Add sweet potatoes, celery,

red pepper and scallions; toss gently.

Season to taste with low sodium salt and pepper.

Cover and refrigerate about 1 hour.

Fold in pecans and sprinkle with chives.

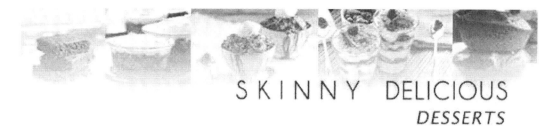

DESSERTS

202. Fabulous Brownie Treats
Ingredients:

1 1/2 cups walnuts

Pinch of low sodium salt

1 tsp vanilla

1/3 cup unsweetened cocoa powder

Instructions:

Add walnuts and low sodium salt to a blender or food processor. Mix until the walnuts are finely ground.

Add the vanilla, and cocoa powder to the blender. Mix well until everything is combined.

With the blender still running, add a couple drops of water at a time to make the mixture stick together.

Using a spatula, transfer the mixture into a bowl. Using your hands, form small round balls, rolling in your palm.

203. Rose Banana Delicious Brownies
Ingredients:

2 red beets, cooked

2 bananas

2 eggs

1/2 cup unsweetened cacao powder

1/3 cup almond flour

1 tsp baking powder

3 tablespoons crushes mixed nuts

Stevia to taste

Instructions:

Combine all ingredients in a food processor, and blend until smooth.

Stir in the nut bits

Pour into a well-greased pan about 8x8 inches

Bake at 325 for about 40 minutes.

204. Pristine Pumpkin Divine

Ingredients:

2 cups blanched almond flour

½ cup flaxseed meal

2 teaspoons ground cinnamon (optional)

Stevia to taste

½ teaspoon low sodium salt

1 egg

1 cup pumpkin puree

1 tablespoon vanilla extract

Instructions:

Mix together the almond flour, flaxseed meal, cinnamon, and low sodium salt

In a separate bowl, whisk the egg, pumpkin and vanilla extract using a rubber spatula.

Gently mix dry and wet ingredients to form a batter being careful not to over mix or the batter will get oily and dense.

Spoon the batter onto a 9-inch pan lined with parchment paper or grease the pan

bake at 350°F until a toothpick inserted into the center comes out clean, approximately 25 minutes.

205. Secret Brownies

Ingredients:

1 c. raw almonds

1/2 c. raw cashews

4-5 Tbs. cocoa powder

1 Tbs. cashew butter

Stevia to taste

Instructions:

Combine all ingredients in the food processor.

Whir until somewhat smooth.

Press into 8×8" glass baking dish.

Chill until ready to serve.

206. Spectacular Spinach Brownies

Ingredients:

1 ¼ cups frozen chopped spinach

6 oz sugar free chocolate

½ cup extra virgin coconut oil

½ cup coconut oil

6 eggs

Stevia to taste

½ cup cocoa powder

1 Tspn vanilla pod

¼ tsp baking soda

½ tsp low sodium salt

½ tsp cream of tartar

pinch cinnamon

Instructions:

Preheat oven to 325F. Line a 9"x13" baking pan with wax paper or use a silicone baking pan.

Melt coconut oil and chocolate together over low heat on the stove top or medium power in the microwave. Add vanilla and stir to incorporate. Let cool.

Mix cocoa powder, baking soda, cream of tartar, low sodium salt and cinnamon.

Blend spinach, egg, together in a food processor or blender, until completely smooth (2-4 minutes).

Add coconut oil to food processor and process until full incorporated.

Add melted chocolate mixture and 3 or 4 drops stevia liquid to egg mixture slowly and processing/blending constantly.

Mix in dry ingredients and process/stir to fully incorporate.

Pour batter into prepared baking pan and spread out with a spatula.

Bake for 40 minutes. Cool completely in pan. Cut into squares. Enjoy!

207. Choco-coco Brownies
Ingredients:

6 Tablespoons of coconut oil

6 ounces of Sugar free Chocolate

4 Tablespoons of Packed Coconut Flour (20g)

¼ cup of Unsweetened Cocoa Powder (30g)

2 Eggs

½ teaspoon of Baking Soda

¼ teaspoon of low sodium salt

Extra coconut oil for pan greasing

Stevia to taste

Instructions:

Preheat the oven to 350F. Grease an 8x8 baking pan and line with parchment paper.

Ensure eggs are at room temperature. You may run them under warm water for about 10 seconds while shelled.

Gently melt the semisweet chocolate and oil in a double boiler. You may use the microwave at 50% heat at 30 second intervals with intermittent stirring.

Stir in unsweetened cocoa powder.

Sift together the superfine coconut flour, baking soda, stevia and low sodium salt.

Beat the eggs and add the dry ingredients. Beat until combined

Add the rest of the wet ingredients and beat until incorporated.

Pour the batter into the lined 8x8 pan.

Bake for 25-30 minutes at 350F until a toothpick inserted into the center of the batter comes out clean.

When done, remove from the oven and let cool in the pan for at least 15 minutes.

208. Coco – Walnut Brownie Bites

Ingredients:

2/3 cup raw walnut halves and pieces

1/3 cup unsweetened cocoa powder

1 tablespoon vanilla extract

1 to 2 tablespoons coconut milk

2/3 cups shredded unsweetened coconut

Instructions:

Pulse coconut in food processor for 30 seconds to a minute to form coconut crumbs. Remove from food processor and set aside.

Add unsweetened cocoa powder and walnuts to food processor, blend until walnuts become fine crumbs, but do not over process or you will get some kind of chocolate walnut butter.

Place in the food processor the cocoa walnut crumbs. Add vanilla. Process until mixture starts to combine.

Add coconut milk. You will know the consistency is right when the dough combines into a ball in the middle of the food processor.

If dough is too runny add a tablespoon or more cocoa powder to bring it back to a dough like state.

Transfer dough to a bowl and cover with plastic wrap. Refrigerate for at least 2 hours. Cold dough is much easier to work with. I left my dough in the fridge over night. You could put it in the freezer if you need to speed the process up.

Roll the dough balls in coconut crumbs, pressing the crumbs gently into the ball. Continue until all dough is gone.

209. Best Ever Banana Surprise Cake
Ingredients:

Bottom Fruit Layer:

2 tbsps coconut oil, melted

1 small banana, sliced, or ¼ cup blueberries for low carb version

2 tbsps walnut pieces * optional, can omit for nut free.

Stevia to taste

1 tsp ground cinnamon.

Top Cake Layer:

2 eggs, beaten.

Stevia to taste

¼ cup unsweetened coconut milk, or unsweetened almond milk.

1 tsp organic GF vanilla extract, or 1 tsp ground vanilla bean

½ tsp baking soda.

1 tsp apple cider vinegar.

1 small banana, mashed, or ¼ cup blueberries for lower carb version.

⅓ cup coconut flour

Instructions:

Preheat oven to 350 F, and lightly grease a 9 inch cake pan.

Place 2 tbsps coconut oil into cake pan, and put pan into preheating oven for a couple minutes to melt butter or oil. Once melted, make sure butter or oil is evenly distributed all over the bottom of the pan.

Sprinkle 2-4 drops stevia sweetener all over the melted oil.

Sprinkle 1 tsp cinnamon on top of sweetener layer.

Layer banana slices or blueberries on top of butter- sweetener layer, as seen in photo above. Add optional walnut pieces to fruit layer. Set aside.

In a large mixing bowl combine all the "top cake layer" ingredients except for the coconut flour. Mix thoroughly, then add the coconut flour and mix well, scraping sides of bowl, and braking up any coconut flour clumps.

Spoon cake batter on top of fruit layer in cake pan

Spread cake batter evenly across entire pan.

Bake for 25 minutes or until top of cake is browned and center is set.

Remove from oven and let cool completely.

Use a butter knife between cake and edge of pan and slide around to loosen cake from pan. Turn cake pan upside down onto a large plate or serving platter.

Slice and serve.

Should be stored in fridge, if serving later.

210. Choco Cookie Delight

Ingredients:

1/2 cup dark chocolate sugar free chips

1/2 cup coconut milk (thick fat from top of can)

2 eggs

1 cup almond flour

pinch of low sodium salt

1/2 teaspoon vanilla extract

1/4 teaspoon baking powder

Vanilla glaze:

1/2 cup coconut butter, liquid

Stevia to taste

1 /2 teaspoon vanilla extract

Chocolate Glaze:

1/2 cup chocolate chips

Stevia powder for decoration

Instructions:

Place a small sauce pan over low heat and melt your chocolate and coconut milk together (only keep the heat on long enough to melt them together)

While melting, place your 2 eggs in a stand mixer with the whisk, or use a hand mixer with the whisk and beat your eggs until they are fluffy, about 1 minute

Add your coconut milk and chocolate to your eggs and mix well

Stir in your almond flour, low sodium salt, vanilla extract and baking powder

Mix well ensuring everything is combined

Pipe your batter into the cookie wells ensuring you fill higher than the halfway point

Remove from the cookie maker, gently insert the sticks and place everything in the freezer for 30-45 minutes

Vanilla Glaze:

Combine your coconut butter, stevia, and vanilla extract in a small glass to make it easy to dip

You can keep this glass in hot water to keep the glaze more liquidy to make the dipping easier

Chocolate Glaze:

Melt your chocolate chips over a double boiler and keep the heat low and them liquid – then spread over cooled cookies!

211. Choco Triple Delight

Ingredients:

Cake:

1 cup almond flour (or 3 oz ground raw pumpkin seeds for nut-free version)

3 tbsp Raw Cacao Powder

1 tbsp coconut flour

1 tsp baking powder

1/2 tsp baking soda

1/8th tsp Stevia

3 tbsp melted Raw Cacao Butter or coconut oil)

Pinch of low sodium salt

1 large pastured egg

2 tbsp coconut milk (or dairy of choice)

1 tsp pure vanilla extract

2 oz 80% cocoa bar, chopped

Top with 2 tbsp chopped nut of choice,

Optional: 1/8th tsp low sodium salt sprinkled on top of cake before baking

Chocolate Drizzle:

2 tbsp coconut cream concentrate, warmed

3 tbsp water (or coconut milk)

3 tbsp Cacao powder

1/2 tbsp pure vanilla extract

Stevia to taste

Instructions:

Preheat oven to 350 degrees F.

Oil the sides and bottom of 8 inch cake pan.

Line the bottom of the pan with parchment paper and set aside.

In a medium bowl, add dry ingredients. Use a sifter to insure that all ingredients are blended well and that there are no lumps.

Add remaining ingredients (except nuts and optional salt) to dry ingredients and mix. Taste for sweetness and adjust if necessary.

Press (or spread with angled spatula) into a 8 inch cake pan. Sprinkle with nuts. Bake for 11-14 minutes.

DO NOT OVER BAKE! Remove from oven and serve warm or allow to cool and top with Chocolate Drizzle.

Chocolate Drizzle:

In a small bowl, blend coconut cream concentrate and water until smooth.

Add cacao powder, vanilla and stevia. Whisk until creamy.

Taste for sweetness and adjust if necessary. Drizzle over the cake.

212. Peach and Almond Cake

Ingredients:

2 whole peaches

300g almond meal

6 eggs

Stevia to taste

1 tsp baking soda

Instructions:

Cover the peaches in water in a saucepan and boil for about 2 hours.

Preheat the oven to 180 degrees Celsius and line the bottom of a 24cm pan with baking paper.

Lightly beat the eggs.

Blend the eggs and peaches (quarter them first) thoroughly in a food processor.

Add the rest of the ingredients to the food processor, again blending thoroughly.

Pour mixture into the lined tin and bake for roughly an hour.

213. Apple Cinnamon Walnut Bonanza

Ingredients:

For the cake:

1 cup almond flour

2 tablespoons coconut flour

Stevia to taste

1 tablespoon cinnamon

1 teaspoon baking soda

1/4 teaspoon low sodium salt

1 tablespoon coconut butter, plus more for greasing the pan

2 eggs

1/2 cup cream from a can of refrigerated coconut milk

1 teaspoon vanilla

1 cup grated apple (about 1 large apple)

For the topping:

1 1/2 cups walnuts (or pecans, if you prefer)

1/2 cup almond flour

4 tablespoons melted coconut butter

Stevia to taste

1 tablespoon cinnamon

pinch low sodium salt

Instructions:

Preheat your oven to 350° and grease a 8 x 8 baking dish.

Make the topping: pulse the walnuts in a food processor 10-12 times or until they are course crumbs. Add the remaining ingredients and pulse 2-3 more times until combined. Set aside.

Wipe out and dry the bowl of your food processor and add your dry **cake** ingredients. (almond flour through low sodium salt) Pulse a few times to mix.

Cut the tablespoon of butter into smaller chunks and add it to the dry ingredients. Pulse 8-10 times or until it's cut in to the dry ingredients, similar to if you were making a pie crust.

In a small bowl, mix your wet cake ingredients (eggs through vanilla) and whisk until well combined. Stir in grated apple.

Add to the food processor and mix until combined. Scrape down the sides once or twice to make sure it's well mixed.

Pour into the prepared baking dish and sprinkle the topping over, as evenly as you can.

Bake for 30-35 minutes, or until a toothpick inserted into the center comes out clean.

Allow to cool, and enjoy!

214. Chestnut- Cacao Cake
Ingredients:

100g (1 cup + 1 heaping tablespoon) chestnut flour

50g (1/2 cup) ground almonds (almond flour)

3 eggs, separate

1/2 teaspoon cream of tartar

35g (1/2 cup) raw cacao powder

Stevia to taste

3/4 cup coconut milk

1/2 teaspoon baking soda

Crushed chesnuts

Instructions:

Preheat oven to 180C fan (350F).

Grease a pie/tart pan.

In a clean mixing bowl, beat the egg whites and cream of tartar until stiff peaks form. Set aside.

In another mixing bowl, cream the egg yolks, chestnut flour, ground almonds, stevia, raw cacao, baking soda and coconut milk.

Fold in the egg whites and blend until the white is no longer showing.

Pour into the pie/tart mold.

Sprinkle with crushed chestnuts, if desired.

Bake for 35-40 minutes on the middle rack.

215. Extra Dark Choco Delight

Ingredients:

1 egg

½ very ripe avocado

¼ cup full fat canned coconut milk

2 tbsp cacao powder

1 tbsp carob powder

pinch low sodium salt

pinch cinnamon

1 scoop vanilla flavored hemp protein powder

10g raw hazelnuts

2 tbsp unsweetened shredded coconut

Instructions:

Add the egg, avocado and coconut milk to a small food processor and process until very smooth and process until very smooth and creamy.

Add cacao powder, carob powder, low sodium salt, cinnamon and protein powder and process again until well combined and creamy.

Add hazelnuts and shredded coconut and give a few extra spins until the hazelnuts are reduced to tiny little pieces.

Serve immediately or refrigerate until ready to serve.

Garnish with a little dollop of coconut cream and cacao nibs or shredded coconut and crushed hazelnuts.

This will keep in the refrigerator for a few days in an airtight container.

216. Nut Butter Truffles
Ingredients:

5 tablespoons sunflower seed butter

1 tablespoon coconut oil

2 teaspoons vanilla extract

¾ cup almond flour

1 tablespoon flaxseed meal

pinch of low sodium salt

¼ cup sugar free dark chocolate chips

1 tablespoon cacao butter

chopped almonds (optional)

Instructions:

Add sunflower seed butter, coconut oil, vanilla, almond flour, flaxseed meal and low sodium salt to a large bowl. Please note that you may find a thin layer of oil in the sunflower seed butter jar that separates from the butter and rises to the top. Be sure to mix oil and butter together before scooping into bowl.

Using your hands mix until all ingredients are incorporated (I like using gloves when mixing so the oils from my skin do not get into the mixture)

Roll the dough into 1-inch balls and place them on a sheet of parchment paper and refrigerate for 30 minutes (using 2 teaspoons for each truffle will yield about 14 truffles)

Melt the chocolate chips in a double boiler along with the cacao butter

Dip each truffle in the melted chocolate, one at the time, and place them back on the pan with parchment paper

Top with chopped almonds and refrigerate until the chocolate is firm

217. Fetching Fudge

Ingredients:

1 cup coconut butter

1/4 cup coconut oil

1/4 cup cocoa

1/4 cup cocoa powder + 1 Tbsp

Stevia to taste

1 tsp vanilla

Instructions:

In the pot, gently melt the cocoa butter on low (number 2)

When it is half melted add the butter, the coconut oil and the coconut spread and gently mix with the whisk as it melts

Add vanilla, and stevia and whisk in well

Add the cocoa powder and whisk in well

Be sure to take the pot off the heat when the fat is melted and keep whisking until it is smooth and all the lumps are out — you don't want to overheat this

Pour into the 8 x 8 pan that is lined with parchment paper

Refrigerate for 1 – 2 hours

When solid, pull the parchment paper out of the pan, put the block of fudge on a flat surface and cut into small squares

Enjoy! This will melt rather quickly — but it won't last long!

218. Choco – Almond Delights
Ingredients:

1 c. toasted hazelnuts

1 c. raw almonds

2/3 c. raw almond butter

5 Tbs. raw cacao powder (or unsweetened cocoa powder)

1/2 tsp. vanilla extract

1/4 c. unsweetened, shredded coconut

Instructions:

Combine all the ingredients, except for the coconut, in the food processor. Whir until smooth. This will take a few minutes and may require scraping down the sides of the bowl one or more times.

Line a mini muffin tin with plastic wrap. Spoon dollops of the sweet mixture into the lined tin cups and form into "mounds." Freeze until well formed. Remove mounds from plastic and tin and flip for presentation. Sprinkle with shredded coconut.

219. Chococups
Ingredients:

4 eggs

Stevia to taste

1/3 cup coconut flour

1/4 cup cacao powder

1/2 teaspoon baking soda

1/4 cup coconut oil (melted in microwave)

1/4 cup cacao butter (melted in microwave)

For topping:

1 can coconut cream (chilled in fridge overnight)

Cacao nibs to decorate.

Instructions:

Heat oven to 170 degrees Celsius (338F)

Grease 10 muffin pans with coconut oil.

Beat eggs with electric beaters.

Add coconut flour, baking soda and cacao powder.

Beat well and add stevia

Add melted coconut oil, cacao butter and mix.

Spoon mixture into 10 greased muffin pans.

Bake for 12-15 minutes until risen and top springs back.

Cool in pans.

Beat the solid coconut cream with electric beaters until creamy. Add honey to taste if you wish.

Pipe coconut cream onto top of cakes.

220. Choco Coco Cookies

Ingredients:

Stevia powder – 1 teaspoon

1 cup coconut flour

½ cup coconut oil

½ cup coconut milk, (from the can)

2 Teaspoons vanilla extract

¼ Teaspoon low sodium salt

2½ cups finely shredded coconut

1 cup big flake coconut

⅔ cup dark sugar free chocolate chunks or chocolate chips (I used 80% dark chocolate)

Optional: ½ cup almond or cashew butter

Instructions:

In a large saucepan, combine the, coconut oil, and coconut milk. Bring the mixture to a boil, and boil for 2-3 minutes.

Remove from the heat and add the vanilla, low sodium salt, and coconut flour and coconut. Stir to combine. If you're using the almond or cashew butter, mix it in thoroughly. Finally, add the chocolate chunks and combine, stirring as little as possible to keep the chunks intact.

Portion the cookie on a parchment lined baking sheet and let cool. This version of no-bakes takes a full 3-4 hours to fully set up, but you don't have to wait that long because they're really good warm and gooey.

221. Apple Spice Spectacular
Ingredients:

1 cup unsweetened almond butter

Stevia to taste

1 egg

1 tsp baking soda

1/2 tsp low sodium salt

half an apple, diced 1 tsp cinnamon

1/4 tsp ground cloves

1/8 tsp nutmeg

1 tsp fresh ginger, grated on a microplane

Instructions:

Pre-heat oven to 350 degress F.

In a large bowl, combine almond butter, stevia, egg, baking soda, and low sodium salt until well incorporated. Add apple, spices, and ginger and stir to combine.

236

Spoon batter onto a baking sheet (you may have to spread the batter a little to get it into a round shape) about 1-2 inches apart from each other--they'll spread a bit.

Bake about 10 minutes, or until slightly set.

Remove cookies and allow to cool on pan for about 5-10 minutes. Then finish cooling on a cooling rack.

222. Absolute Almond Bites

Ingredients:

1 1/2 cups almond flour

1/4 teaspoon low sodium salt

1/4 teaspoon baking soda (gluten-free, if necessary)

1/8 teaspoon cinnamon

2 tablespoons melted coconut oil

Stevia to taste

1 1/4 teaspoon vanilla extract

1/4 teaspoon almond extract or almond flavoring

12 to 15 whole almonds; sprouted or soaked and dehydrated

Instructions:

Preheat oven to 325°F. Line a baking sheet with parchment paper.

In a medium bowl combine almond flour, low sodium salt, baking soda, and cinnamon. Mix well, breaking up any lumps.

In a small bowl, place coconut oil, vanilla, almond extract or flavoring. Whisk until well combined.

Add wet ingredients to dry ingredients and stir until combined...add stevia

Roll level-tablespoon-sized (using a measuring spoon) portions of dough into balls and place on baking sheet. Flatten slightly with the heel of your hand and press one almond into the center of each cookie.

Bake 15 to 17 minutes or until light golden brown. Allow to cool on baking sheet for a few minutes before transferring to cooling rack.

Store in an airtight container. Can be frozen.

223. Eastern Spice Delights

Ingredients:

1 3/4 cups + 4 tbsp almond meal

1/8 tsp low sodium salt

3/4 tsp ground ginger

3/4 tsp cinnamon

1/4 tsp ground cloves

1/4 tsp cardamom

1/8 tsp nutmeg

1/2 cup coconut oil (in solid form)

Stevia to taste

1 tsp vanilla extract

Instructions:

Preheat oven to 350F.

Combine all the dry ingredients in a large bowl. In a small bowl, mix together the oil, maple syrup, and vanilla until completely blended. Pour the wet ingredients over the dry ingredients and mix well.

Drop the cookie dough on a cookie sheet. It will spread a bit as it cooks (and thus flatten), but not an awful lot.

Bake for 10-12 minutes. These cookies will not look golden when they're done. Makes two dozens.

224. Berry Ice Cream and Almond Delight

Ingredients:

For the Ice Cream:

1 can full fat coconut milk

Stevia to taste

2 tbsp vanilla

1 cup fresh strawberries cut into fourths

For the crisp:

1/3 cup almond flour

3 tbsp sunflower seed butter (or almond butter)

1/2 tsp vanilla

1 tbsp honey

low sodium salt to taste

Instructions:

For the ice cream:

Combine coconut milk and vanilla together in a small saucepan over medium heat and stir until ingredients are well combined (just a few minutes).

Transfer milk mixture to a small bowl and place in the freezer for two hours.

Next, add strawberries to a small saucepan and bring to a low boil.

Turn heat to medium-low and allow to cook until they start breaking down into a sauce-like mixture, leaving small chunks.

Place strawberries in refrigerator while the ice cream hardens.

For the crisp:

Combine all ingredients and mix until you get a "crumble' consistency.

Place crisp in refrigerator until ready to use.

After two hours, place milk mixture into your ice cream maker along with the strawberries and use as directed.

When ice cream is ready, scoop and serve with crisp sprinkled on top.

225. Creamy Caramely Ice Cream

Ingredients:

Delicious Instant Caramel Topping:

2 heaped tablespoons of hulled tahini

Stevia to taste

2 tablespoons of coconut milk

1/2 teaspoon of vanilla

Delicious Instant Ice Cream:

4 frozen bananas, chopped

4 tablespoons coconut milk

1 teaspoon of vanilla

Instructions:

Spoon the tahini and stevia into a cup and stir with a fork to combine. Mix in the coconut milk and vanilla. Refrain from eating it while you make your ice cream.

Place the ingredients into food processor or blender, blend until the mixture is an ice cream consistency.

Spoon the ice cream into bowls, drizzle generously with the caramel topping, sprinkle with low sodium salt if you desire. Enjoy!

226. Cheeky Cherry Ice

Ingredients:

14oz. cans 365 Coconut Milk (Full Fat)

Stevia to taste

1 ½ tsp. vanilla extract

2 cups fresh cherries, pitted and diced

Instructions:

In a large bowl, combine coconut milk, stevia and vanilla and stir well.

Chill for 1-2 hours.

Transfer to ice-cream maker and process according to manufacturer directions.

Add diced cherries to the mixture during the last 5-10 minutes of processing.

227. Choco - Coconut Berry Ice

Ingredients:

Follow recipe of berry ice cream and almond delight for the ice cream only

4 ounces sugar free dark chocolate - 75% cacao content

¼ cup coconut milk

2 cups fresh berries (I used raspberries)

Instructions:

Make the Homemade Coconut Ice Cream,

While the ice cream is freezing in the machine, break the chocolate into pieces and place in a small saucepan.

Add the coconut milk and melt the two together, stirring over low heat.

When the chocolate mixture is completely smooth, pour the chocolate over the ice cream and stir to create 'ripples'. If your ice cream if thoroughly frozen, soften in the fridge for 20 minutes before stirring in the chocolate.

Serve immediately with the fresh berries, or freeze for an additional 3-4 hours for a firmer texture.

228. Creamy Berrie Pie

Ingredients:

Crust:

3 cups almonds

½ Teaspoon cinnamon

½ cup honey

2 Tablespoons coconut oil

1 Tablespoon lemon zest

1 Teaspoon almond extract

A pinch of low sodium salt

Filling:

2 Teaspoons plant-based gelatin, dissolved in 2 Tablespoons hot water

⅓ cup freshly squeezed lemon juice

Stevia to taste

1 can coconut milk, chilled

4 cups blueberries for serving

Instructions:

Place the almonds and cinnamon in a food processor and pulse until your desired texture is reached. I like to leave some bigger pieces for texture. Add the rest of the crust ingredients and pulse until a sticky dough forms. Pat the crust into a pie plate, (use water to keep your hands from sticking to the crust).

For the filling, mix the gelatin and water together. Stir to dissolve and immediately add the lemon juice. If the gelatin gets clumpy, place the mixture over hot water until it melts again. Pour the coconut milk into an electric mixer, add the stevia and whip on high until peaks form, about 15 minutes. Add the gelatin mixture to the whipped cream. Pour the filling into the crust. The filling will seem thin, but don't worry it will set up in the refrigerator.

Chill for at least 4 hours until set, and serve with lots of berries!

229. Peachy Creamy Peaches
Ingredients:

3 medium ripe peaches cut in half with pit removed

1 tsp vanilla

1 can coconut milk, refrigerated

1/4 cup chopped walnuts

Cinnamon (to taste)

Instructions:

Place peaches on the grill with the cut side down first. Grill on medium-low heat until soft, about 3-5 minutes on each side.

Scoop cream off the top of the can of chilled coconut milk. Whip together coconut cream and vanilla with handheld mixer. Drizzle over each peach. Top with cinnamon and chopped walnuts to garnish.

230. Spiced Apple Bake
Ingredients:

2 apples of your choice

1/4 cup walnuts

1/4 tablespoon nutmeg

1/4 tablespoon cinnamon

1/4 tablespoon ground cloves

Instructions:

Preheat oven to 350 degrees Fahrenheit.

Slice the very top and very bottom off of each apple. (The top allows for more room to stuff with goodies, the bottom allows the apples to soak up all the nice sauce).

Core both apples to the bottom, but not all the way through.

Mix spices, walnuts, and raisins in a small bowl.

Pour half of the spice mixture into each apple.

Place on baking sheet and bake 20-25 minutes, or until apples are soft. I like to pour any remaining sauce mixture into the bottom of the pan so the apples can soak up the flavors.

231. Sexy Dessert Pan
Ingredients:

Crust:

1 1/2 cups pecans

3/4 cup dates

4 tbsp coconut oil

Second Layer:

2/3 cup cashew butter

1/3 cup palm shortening

2 tsp apple cider vinegar

1/2 tsp lemon juice

Pinch low sodium salt

Third Layer:

1 cup coconut flour

1 cup coconut milk

Stevia to taste

1 tsp vanilla extract

Fourth Layer:

1/2 cup coconut milk

1/2 cup coconut butter

1/2 cup cacao powder

2 tbsp honey

Fifth Layer:

1/2 cup coconut butter

1/4 cup coconut milk

Stevia to taste

Sixth Layer:

Grated dark sugar free chocolate, at least 80% cocoa

Instructions:

To make the crust, roughly chop the pecans then pit and chop the dates. Load both into a food processor and pulse until ground but still crumbly. Transfer to a bowl and work in the coconut oil, then press the sticky mixture into a single smooth layer at the bottom of a square 8x8 cake pan.

Transfer to the refrigerator to chill while you begin the second layer. To make the second layer, combine its ingredients very well in a medium mixing bowl. Spoon over the chilled crust, smoothing as much as possible with the back of a spoon. Place the pan back in the fridge.

To make the third layer, mix its ingredients together in a mixing bowl and then spoon over the chilled, hardened second layer. Smooth as much as possible, then chill.

Add the fourth layer by combining its ingredients and then layering it into the pan in the same way as the previous layers.

For the fifth layer, mix the coconut shortening, coconut milk and stevia with a hand mixer until very smooth and spoon over the chilled fourth layer.

Before placing the pan back into the refrigerator after adding the fifth layer, grate very dark chocolate over the top to the depth of your preference. Chill the pan for an additional half hour or more, then slice with a sharp knife and serve.

Notes:

The layers may seem fiddly but the technique is so simple once you're in the thick of it: just mix the ingredients, spoon into the pan and chill!

232. Pretty Pumpkin Delights
Ingredients:

For Crust:

1 cup hazelnuts (preferably soaked and dehydrated for better digestion)

1/2 cup raw pumpkin seeds (preferably soaked and dehydrated for better digestion)

1 TBS coconut oil

2 pinches of low sodium salt

Stevia to taste

For Filling:

1 cup cooked pumpkin puree

1/2 cup coconut

2 TBS coconut oil

Stevia to taste

1/2 tsp vanilla extract

1/4 tsp cinnamon powder

1/4 tsp ginger powder

1/8 tsp allspice

1/8 tsp clove powder

For Chocolate Drizzle:

2 TBS coconut butter

2 TBS coconut oil

2 TBS raw cacao (or unsweetened cocoa)

Stevia to taste

a pinch or 2 of low sodium salt

Instructions:

To Make the crust: Line mini muffin tins with unbleached mini paper liners. Process all crust ingredients in a food processor until well combined and resembles a coarse flour. Spoon 1 and 1/2 tsp of mixture into each of the 24 mini cups. Use your thumb to press down mixture firmly to create a solid bottom layer for these cute little yummies. Place in freezer to harden.

To make filling: Melt coconut butter and coconut oil in a double boiler. Remove from heat and add rest of filling ingredients. Go ahead and mix it up real good here until creamy smooth. Remove crusts from freezer and spoon about 3/4 TBS of filling over your prepared crusts. Return to freezer to harden, at least 2 hours.

To make chocolate drizzle: Once mini bites have hardened, gently melt coconut butter and coconut oil in a double boiler. Remove from heat and add rest of drizzle ingredients. Allow to cool slightly to thicken. Pour into small plastic bag, cut a TINY hole in the corner, and drizzle over treats in any fashion that you want.

Now it's time to enjoy these amazing delights. Store leftovers in freezer as they are best cold. (That is, if there are any leftovers. Ours got dusted off in one day.)

233. Macadamia Pineapple Bonanza

Ingredients:

Crust:

½ cup almond flour

4 tablespoons raw cacao powder

⅓ cup macadamia nuts

½ teaspoon vanilla extract

Stevia to taste

1½ teaspoons coconut oil, melted

Filling:

2 eggs

1 cup fresh pineapple, chopped

1⅓ cup shredded coconut, unsweetened

1 tablespoon fresh lime juice

1 tablespoon vanilla extract

Stevia to taste

½ cup almond flour

A pinch of low sodium salt

Instructions:

Crust:

In a large bowl, mix the almond flour and cacao powder.

Chop the macadamia nuts in a food processor and add it to the bowl.

Add vanilla extract and coconut oil to the dry mixture and using your hands, mix to combine ingredients.

Spread the mixture evenly on the bottom of an 8x8-inch pan lined with parchment paper. Be sure to use one large piece of paper covering the entire pan that overlaps on all four sides.

Filing:

In a large bowl beat the 2 eggs

Mix in the pineapple, 1 cup of shredded coconut (reserve the remaining ⅓ cup for the top), lime juice, vanilla and stevia.

Gently mix in the almond flour and low sodium salt with rubber spatula.

Pour mixture over the crust and sprinkle top with remaining shredded coconut.

Bake at 350°F for approximately 20 minutes or until the top starts to brown and the pineapple/coconut layer is firm.

Set pan on a wire rack and allow it to cool before cutting into squares. Store in the refrigerator.

234. Lemonny Lemon Delights
Ingredients:

Crust:

1 cup almond flour

1/4 cup almond butter

Stevia to taste

1 tbsp coconut butter

1 tsp vanilla

1/2 tsp baking powder

1/4 tsp low sodium salt

Filling:

3 eggs

Stevia to taste

1/4 cup lemon juice

2 1/2 tbsp coconut flour

1 tbsp lemon zest, finely grated

Pinch of low sodium salt

Instructions:

Preheat oven to 350.

Coat 9×9 baking dish with coconut oil or butter.

Combine all crust ingredients in food processor until a "crumble" forms.

Press crust evenly into the bottom of pan.

Using a fork, prick a few holes into crust.

Bake for 10 minutes.

While crust is baking, combine all filling ingredients in a food processor until well incorporated.

When done, remove crust from oven and pour filling evenly over top.

Continue to bake for 15-20 minutes, or until filling is set, but still has a little jiggle.

Cool completely on wire rack. (You can also chill in the fridge if desired, to further set the filling).

235. Gluten Free Banana Nut Bread

Ingredients:

3 bananas, mashed, or 1 cup

3 eggs

1/2 cup almond butter

1/4 cup coconut oil, melted

1 tsp vanilla extract

1/2 cup almond flour

1/2 cup coconut flour

2 tsp cinnamon

1 tsp baking soda

1/4 tsp low sodium salt

1/2 cup chopped walnuts

Instructions:

Preheat the oven to 350 degrees F. Line a loaf pan with parchment paper. In a large bowl, add the mashed bananas, eggs, almond butter, coconut oil, and vanilla. Use a hand blender to combine.

In a separate bowl, mix together the almond flour, coconut flour, cinnamon, baking soda, and low sodium salt. Blend the dry ingredients into the wet mixture, scraping down the sides with a spatula. Fold in the walnuts.

Pour the batter into the loaf pan in an even layer. Bake for 50-60 minutes, until a toothpick inserted into the center comes out clean. Place the bread on a cooling rack and allow to cool before slicing.

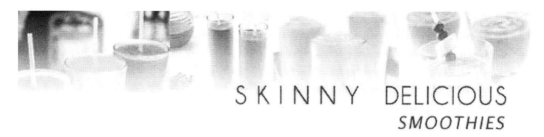

SKINNY DELICIOUS
SMOOTHIES

SMOOTHIES

236. Gorgeous Berry Smoothie
Ingredients:

½ cup frozen blueberries or 1 cup fresh blueberries

15 oz coconut milk

Stevia to taste

1 scoop of hemp protein

¼ teaspoon cinnamon (optional)

Instructions:

Place all ingredients into a blender.

Blend until mixed thoroughly.

Serve right away.

237. Tempting Coconut Berry Smoothie
Ingredients:

½ Cup Frozen Blackberries

½ Frozen Banana

1 Teaspoon Chia Seeds

¼ Inch Piece Of Fresh Ginger

½ Cup Almond

Coconut Milk

1 scoop of HEMP protein

2 Tablespoons Toasted Coconut

Instructions:

Combine all the ingredients in a blender and process until smooth.

238. Voluptuous Vanilla Hot Drink
Ingredients:

3 cups unsweetened almond milk (or 1 1/2 cup full fat coconut milk + 1 1/2 cups of

water)
Stevia to taste

1 scoop of hemp protein

1/2 Tbsp. ground cinnamon (or more to taste)

1/2 Tbsp. vanilla extract

Instructions:

Place the almond milk into a pitcher. Place ground cinnamon, hemp, anilla extract in a small saucepan over medium high heat. Heat until the pure liquid stevia is just melted and then pour the pure liquid stevia mixture into the pitcher.

Stir until the pure liquid stevia is well combined with the almond milk. Place the pitcher in the fridge and allow to chill for at least two hours. Stir well before serving.

239. Almond Butter Smoothies
Ingredients:

1 scoop of hemp protein

1 Tablespoon natural almond butter

1 cup of hemp milk

1 banana, preferably frozen for a creamier shake

few ice cubes

Instructions:

Blend all ingredients together and enjoy!

240. Choco Walnut Delight
Ingredients:

1 scoop Hemp Protein

30g dark sugar free chocolate broken up.

50g walnuts chopped/crushed (depending on desired texture)

250ml hemp milk or nut milk alternative

A handful of ice cubes, the more you use the thicker it will be.

Instructions:

Blend everything together in a strong blender until thoroughly processed, and enjoy!

Makes 2, and can be stored in the fridge overnight.

241. Raspberry Hemp Smoothie
Ingredients:

1 cup hemp milk or milk alternative

1/2 cup raspberries (fresh or frozen)

2 tablespoons hemp protein powder

Stevia to taste

3 to 4 ice cubes

Instructions:

Add ingredients to a blender and blend until smooth.

242. Choco Banana Smoothie
Ingredients:

1 cup milk or milk alternative

2 peeled frozen bananas

4 ice cubes

2 tablespoons hulled hemp seed

2 tablespoons hemp protein powder

1 tablespoons organic cocoa powder

5-7 drops liquid stevia to sweeten

1/4 teaspoon cinnamon

1/4 teaspoon vanilla

Instructions:

Put all ingredients into blender. Blend until smooth.

243. Blueberry Almond Smoothie
Ingredients:

1 c almond milk
1 c frozen unsweetened blueberries
1 tbsp cold-pressed organic flaxseed oil
2 tbsps hemp protein powder

Instructions:

Combine milk and blueberries in blender, and blend for 1 minute.

Transfer to glass, and stir in flaxseed oil.

244. Hazelnut Butter and Banana Smoothie
Ingredients:

½ c nut milk

½ c hemp milk

2 Tbsp creamy natural unsalted hazelnut butter

¼ very ripe banana

stevia drops to taste

4 ice cubes

2 tsp hemp protein powder

Instructions:

Combine ingredients in a blender. Process until smooth.

Pour into a tall glass and serve.

245. Vanilla Blueberry Smoothie
Ingredients:

2 cups hemp milk

1 c fresh blueberries

Handful of ice OR 1 cup frozen blueberries

1 Tbsp flaxseed oil (MUFA)

2 tsp hemp protein powder

Instructions:

Combine milk, and fresh blueberries plus ice (or frozen blueberries) in a blender.

Blend for 1 minute, transfer to a glass, and stir in flaxseed oil.

246. Chocolate Raspberry Smoothie
Ingredients:

1 cup almond milk

¼ c chocolate chips-sugar free

1 c fresh raspberries

2 tsp hemp protein powder

Handful of ice OR 1 cup frozen raspberries

Instructions:

COMBINE ingredients in a blender.

Blend for 1 minute, transfer to a glass, and eat with a spoon.

247. Peach Smoothie
Ingredients:

1 cup hemp milk

1 c frozen unsweetened peaches

2 tsp cold-pressed organic flaxseed oil (MUFA)

2 tsp hemp protein powder

Instructions:

PLACE milk and frozen, unsweetened peaches in blender and blend for 1 minute.

Transfer to glass, and stir in flaxseed oil.

248. Zesty Citrus Smoothie
Ingredients:

1 cup almond milk

half cup lemon juice

1 med orange peeled, cleaned, and sliced into sections

Handful of ice

1 tbsp flaxseed oil

2 tsps hemp protein powder

Instructions:

COMBINE milk, lemon juice, orange, and ice in a blender.

Blend for 1 minute, transfer to a glass, and stir in flaxseed oil.

249. Apple Smoothie

Ingredients:

½ cup hemp milk

1 cup hemp milk

1 tsp apple pie spice

1 med apple peeled and chopped

2 Tbsp cashew butter

Handful of ice

2 tsp hemp protein powder

Instructions:

COMBINE ingredients in a blender.

Blend for 1 minute, transfer to a glass, and eat with a spoon.

250. Pineapple Smoothie

Ingredients:

1 cup almond milk

4 oz fresh pineapple

Handful of ice

2 tbsps hemp protein powder

1 tbsp cold-pressed organic flaxseed oil

Instructions:

PLACE milk, canned pineapple in blender, add of ice, and whip for 1 minute.

Transfer to glass and stir in flaxseed oil.

251. Strawberry Smoothie

Ingredients:

1 cup almond milk

1 c frozen, unsweetened strawberries

2 tbsps hemp protein powder

2 tbsps cold-pressed organic flaxseed oil

Instructions:

COMBINE milk and strawberries in blender.

Blend, transfer to glass, and stir in flaxseed oil.

252. Pineapple Coconut Deluxe Smoothie

Ingredients:

1 C pineapple chunks

1 C coconut milk

1/2 C pineapple juice

1 ripe banana

1/2 – 3/4 C ice cubes

Pure liquid stevia to taste

1 tablespoon hemp protein powder

Instructions:

In a blender, combine the pineapple chunks, coconut milk, banana, ice and pure liquid stevia.

Puree until smooth.

Pour into 2 large glasses.

Garnish with a pineapple wedge if desired.

253. Divine Vanilla Smoothie

Ingredients:

1 cup coconut or almond milk

¼ cup almond butter

1 tsp vanilla paste, (or vanilla extract)

2 cups ice

Sweet Leaf Stevia Vanilla Creme, to taste

Vanilla hemp Protein Powder – 1 tablespoon

Instructions:

Add all ingredients except ice to blender. Puree well.

Add ice and blend until ice is all crushed and smoothie is well blended and smooth.

Pour into two glasses and serve immediately.

NOTES
Add more or less ice to make the smoothie thinner or thicker consistency.
Vanilla hemp protein powder would be great to add for a post workout smoothie!

254. Coco Orange Delish Smoothie

Ingredients:

1/2 cup fresh squeezed orange juice (I used 1 1/2 oranges)

1 tablespoon hemp protein powder

1/2 cup full fat coconut milk from the can (not the box!)

1 teaspoon vanilla

1/2 -1 cup crushed ice

Instructions:

Add all ingredients to a blender.

Blend until smooth and add ice as needed to get the consistency you like.

255. Baby Kale Pineapple Smoothie

Ingredients:

1 cup almond milk

1/2 cup frozen pineapple

1 cup Kale

1 tablespoon hemp protein powder

Instructions:

Place the almond milk, pineapple, and greens in the blender and blend until smooth.

256. Sumptuous Strawberry Coconut Smoothie

Ingredients:

1 cup coconut milk

1 frozen banana, sliced

2 cups frozen strawberries

1 teaspoon vanilla extract

1 tablespoon hemp protein powder

Instructions:

Add all ingredients to blender and blend until smooth.

257. Blueberry Bonanza Smoothies

Ingredients:

1/4 cup canned coconut or almond milk

1/2 cup water

1 medium banana, sliced

1 cup frozen blueberries

1 tablespoon raw almonds

Instructions:

Add coconut milk, water, banana, blueberries and almonds to blender container.

Cover and blend until smooth. Pour into 2 glasses.

258. Divine Peach Coconut Smoothie
Ingredients:

1 cup full fat coconut milk, chilled

1 cup ice

2 large fresh peaches, peeled and cut into chunks

fresh lemon zest, to taste

1 tablespoon hemp protein powder

Instructions:

Add coconut milk, ice and peaches blender. Using a zester, add a few gratings of fresh lemon zest.

Blend on high speed until smooth.

259. Tantalizing Key Lime Pie Smoothie
Ingredients:

1 cup coconut milk

1 cup ice

1/2 avocado

zest and juice of 2 limes

Pure liquid stevia to taste

1 tablespoon hemp protein powder

Instructions:

Add all ingredients to Vitamix or blender and blend until smooth.

260. High Protein and Nutritional Delish Smoothie

Ingredients:

1 cup almond milk

1/2 Avocado

4 Strawberries

1/2 Bananas (Very ripe)

1/2 cup Raw Kale or spinach

1/4 cup Carrot or 100 % Orange Juice (legal) (water can be subbed)

1 cup Coconut Yogurt..or almond milk)

1 tablespoon hemp protein powder

Instructions:

Add everything to your blender, More water or ice can be added to help with your preferred texture/thickness.

261. Pineapple Protein Smoothie

Ingredients:

1 cup (135g) pineapple chunks

1 cup (200g) coconut milk (fresh or tinned)

½ med (65g) banana

¼ cup (65g) ice cubes

¼ tsp vanilla bean powder

pinch low sodium salt

1 tablespoon hemp protein powder

Instructions:

Peel pineapple and chop into small chunks.

Put everything into a high speed blender and blend until smooth.

262. Raspberry Coconut Smoothie

Ingredients:

½ - 1 cup coconut milk (depending on how thick you like it)

1 medium banana, peeled sliced and frozen

2 teaspoons coconut extract (optional)

1 cup frozen raspberries

1 tablespoon hemp protein powder

optional: shredded coconut flakes, and stevia to taste

Instructions:

Add coconut milk, frozen banana slices and coconut extract to your blender.

Pulse 1-2 minutes until smooth.

Add frozen raspberries and continue to pulse until smooth.

Pour into your serving glass, top with a couple of raspberries and a little shredded coconut, and enjoy!

263. Ginger Carrot Protein Smoothie

Ingredients:

3/4 cup carrot juice

1 tablespoon hemp protein powder

1 tablespoon hulled hemp seeds

1/2 apple

3 to 4 ice cubes

1/2 inch piece fresh ginger

Instructions:

Add to a blender and blend until smooth.

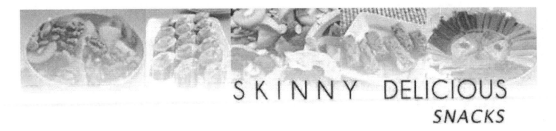

SKINNY DELICIOUS
SNACKS

SNACKS

264. Delish Banana Nut Muffins

Ingredients:

4 bananas, mashed with a fork (the more ripe, the better)

4 eggs

1/2 cup almond butter

2 tbsp coconut oil, melted

1 tsp vanilla

1/2 cup coconut flour

2 tsp cinnamon

1/2 tsp nutmeg

1 tsp baking powder

1 tsp baking soda

1/4 tsp low sodium salt

Instructions:

Preheat oven to 350 degrees F. Line a muffin tin with cups. In a large bowl, add bananas, eggs, almond butter, coconut oil, and vanilla. Using a hand blender, blend to combine.

Add in the coconut flour, cinnamon, nutmeg, baking powder, baking soda, and low sodium salt. Blend into the wet mixture, scraping down the sides with a spatula. Distribute the batter evenly into the lined muffin tins, filling each about two-thirds of the way full.

Bake for 20-25 minutes, until a toothpick comes out clean. Serve warm or store in the refrigerator in a resealable bag.

265. Delightful Cinnamon Apple Muffins

Ingredients:

1 cup unsweetened applesauce

4 eggs

1/4 cup coconut oil, melted

1 tsp vanilla

Stevia to taste

1/2 cup coconut flour

2 tsp cinnamon

1 tsp baking powder

1 tsp baking soda

1/4 tsp low sodium salt

Instructions:

Preheat oven to 350 degrees F. Line a muffin tin with liners. In a large bowl, add applesauce, eggs, coconut oil, stevia, and vanilla. Stir to combine.

Stir in the coconut flour, cinnamon, baking powder, baking soda, and low sodium salt. Distribute the batter evenly into the lined muffin tins, filling each about two-thirds of the way full.

Bake for 15-20 minutes, until a toothpick inserted into the center comes out clean. Serve warm or store in the refrigerator in a resealable bag.

266. Healthy Breakfast Bonanza Muffins

Ingredients:

8 eggs

1 cup diced broccoli

1 cup diced onion

1 cup diced mushrooms

low sodium salt and pepper, to taste

This recipe makes 8 muffins.

Instructions:

Preheat oven to 350 degrees F.

Dice all vegetables. You can add more or less of any of them, but keep the overall portion of vegetables the same for best results.

In a large mixing bowl, whisk together eggs, vegetables, low sodium salt, and pepper.

Pour mixture into a greased muffin pan, the mixture should evenly fill 8 muffin cups.

Bake 18-20 minutes, or until a toothpick inserted in the middle comes out clean.

Serve and enjoy! Leftovers can be saved in the refrigerator throughout the week.

267. Perfect Pumpkin Seeds

Ingredients:

1 cup of pumpkin (only seeds)

2 teaspoons of olive oil

1 tablespoon of chili powder (you may adjust it as per the taste you like)

1 teaspoon low sodium salt

Instructions:

Heat the pan (medium high heat) and place the pumpkin seeds.

After 3 to 5 minutes, you will hear the seeds making a crackling noise (some will even pop). You need to stir frequently.

Remove the pan and mix the seeds in olive oil, then low sodium salt and chili powder. Let it cool and then serve.

268. Gorgeous Spicy Nuts

Ingredients:

2/3 cup of each (almonds, pecans and walnuts)

1 teaspoon of chili powder

½ teaspoon of cumin

½ teaspoon of black

pepper (ground)

½ teaspoon low sodium salt

1 tables

Instructions:

Heat the pan on medium heat and place the nuts and toast them until lightly browned.

Prepare the spice mixture, while the nuts are toasting.

Mix cumin, chili, low sodium salt and black pepper in a bowl and add the nuts (after coating it with olive oil).

269. Krunchy Yummy Kale Chips

Ingredients:

1 bunch of kale, washed and dried

2 tbsp olive oil

low sodium salt to taste

Instructions:

Preheat oven to 300 degrees. Remove the center stems and either tear or cut up the leaves.

Toss the kale and olive oil together in a large bowl; sprinkle with low sodium salt. Spread on a baking sheet

Bake at 300 degrees for 15 minutes or until crisp.

270. Delicious Cinnamon Apple Chips

Ingredients:

1-2 apples

1 tsp cinnamon

Instructions:

Preheat oven to 200 degrees.

Using a sharp knife or mandolin, slice apples thinly. Discard seeds. Prepare a baking sheet with parchment paper and arrange apple slices on it without overlapping. Sprinkle cinnamon over apples.

Bake for approximately 1 hour, then flip. Continue baking for 1-2 hours, flipping occasionally, until the apple slices are no longer moist. Store in airtight container.

271. Gummy Citrus Snack

Ingredients:

3/4 cup lemon juice, freshly squeezed* and ¼ cup apple juice freshly squeezed

4 Tbsp. good quality vegetarian gelatin

3 Tbsp. liquid stevia

1/4 tsp. ginger (freshly grated with a microplane or ground)

1/4 tsp. turmeric (freshly grated with a microplane or ground)

Instructions:

In a small saucepan, whisk together citrus juice, and gelatin until there are no lumps. Heat the liquid over low heat until liquid is warmed and gelatin is completely dissolved.

Remove from heat and stir in liquid stevia, ginger and turmeric with a spoon.

Pour into a casserole dish*.

Refrigerate until liquid is set (at least 30 minutes).

Serve cold or at room temperature.

272. Skinny Delicious Energy Bars

Ingredients:

1 medium, banana

1/4 cup nuts (I used unsalted cashews)

1/4 cup seeds (I used sunflower seeds, or sub for more nuts)

1/4 cup hemp protein powder

2 tbsp coconut flour

1/2 cup almond flour

Instructions:

In a bowl, mash the banana well with a fork or other handy utensil. It doesn't have to be perfect.

Add almond flour and coconut flour and mix well.

Add in your mix-ins and stir well.

Grease a small pan (I used a meatloaf pan and it was perfect) with walnut oil and pour mixture in, pressing down where needed to evenly distribute throughout.

Bake on around 275 for 30-40 minutes, or until the edges start to brown.

Take out the loaf, and cut into cute bars or squares.

Power up as needed! And store in the fridge after a day.

273. Divine Butternut Chips

Ingredients:

1 medium butternut squash (400g / 14.1 oz)

2 tbsp extra virgin coconut oil

1 tsp gingerbread spice mix (~ ½ tsp cinnamon, pinch nutmeg, ginger, cloves and allspice)

pinch low sodium salt (or more in case you don't use stevia and prefer the chips salty)

optional: 3-6 drops liquid Stevia extract

Instructions:

Preheat the oven to 125 C / 250 F. Peel the butternut squash and slice thinly on a mandolin. If you are using a knife, make sure the slices are no more than 1/8 inch (1/4 cm) thin. Place in a bowl.

In a small bowl, mix melted coconut oil, gingerbread spice mix and stevia.

Pour the oil mixture over the butternut squash and mix well to allow it everywhere.

Arrange the slices close to each other on a baking tray lined with parchment paper or a rack or an oven chip tray (you will need at least 2 of them).

Place in the oven and cook for about 1.5 hour or until crispy (the exact time depends on how thick the chips are).

274. Outstanding Orange Skinny Snack
Ingredients:

1 T. vanilla extract

½ t. natural orange flavor

Pinch low sodium salt

1 ½ t. liquid stevia to taste

8 T. vegetarian gelatin

1 can coconut milk

1 ½ C. water

Instructions:

Heat water and coconut milk over low heat until simmering.

Continue on low heat, slowly adding in each tablespoon of gelatin, whisking the entire time.

Add remaining ingredients and whisk until any clumps of gelatin are gone.

Pour into molds, and pour remaining liquid into 8X8 glass pan.

Put in fridge until solid. ...should pop out easily once hardened.

275. Spicy Pumpkin Seed Bonanza

Ingredients:

1 1/2 cups pumpkin seeds,

3 jalapeño peppers, sliced

3 tablespoons olive oil

low sodium salt and paprika, to taste

Instructions:

Preheat the oven to 350°F

Spread pumpkin seeds out on a rimmed baking sheet.

Add olive oil and low sodium salt and stir pumpkin seeds with your hands to combine.

Lay slices of jalapeño peppers on top of seeds.

Sprinkle paprika over the top of everything, generously.

Bake for 10 minutes.

Use a spatula to move the seeds and peppers around. Bake for another 5 minutes.

Move mixture around some more and bake for a final 5 minutes.

Remove tray from oven and let everything rest for 15-30 minutes to let the jalapeño-ness soak into the seeds.

Store in an airtight container...if you don't finish them all in one sitting.

276. Delectable Chocolate-Frosted Doughnuts

Ingredients:

For the doughnuts:

1 tbsp water, separated into

1/2 tablespoons

3 eggs

1 tsp vanilla

1/4 cup coconut flour

1/4 cup coconut oil, melted

1 tbsp cinnamon

1/4 tsp baking soda

low sodium salt to taste

For the frosting:

1/2 cup sugar free dairy free

Chocolate Chips

1 tbsp coconut oil

Instructions:

Turn on donut hole maker (You could also make these into regular donuts and cook at 350 for about 15 or so minutes).

Combine eggs, and vanilla in a food processor until well combined.

Add in the rest of the ingredients and continue to process until all ingredients are incorporated.

Add appropriate amount of batter to donut hole maker and use as instructed (Mine took about 3 or so minutes for each batch, but this will vary for different types).

While your donuts are baking, prepare the frosting by combing chocolate chips and coconut oil over LOW heat until melted.

Once donuts are completely cooled, dip each in frosting with a toothpick or skewer and completely cover, tapping off excess frosting. (I used a longer skewer stick and placed them standing up in a cup to harden, but if you aren't concerned with appearance, you can dip them with a fork or spoon, even, and just place them on a plate).

Place donuts in refrigerator to completely harden (about 1 hour).

277. Eggplant Divine

Ingredients:

1 large eggplant (about 1 pound)

1/2 cup olive oil

4 tablespoons balsamic vinegar

2 tablespoons pure liquid stevia

1/2 teaspoon paprika

low sodium salt

Instructions:

Wash eggplant and slice into thin strips. For ease in snacking you can cut long strips in half crosswise. Leave full-length for a more bacon-like appearance.

In a large bowl whisk together oil, vinegar, stevia, and paprika. Place strips in the mixture a few at a time, turning to make sure each is completely coated. If you run short of marinade, add a little more oil and stir it in with your hands.

Marinate 2 hours. Then, place strips on baking sheets

To dry in the oven: Line one or two rimmed baking sheets with parchment paper. Lay strips on sheets, close together but not overlapping. Sprinkle on a little low sodium salt (you don't need much). Place in oven on lowest setting for 10 to 12 hours (ovens' lowest setting varies, thus drying time will vary) or until dry and fairly crisp, turning strips partway through. Check occasionally, and if any oil pools on the sheets, blot with a paper towel.

278. Choco Apple Nachos

Ingredients:

apples

fresh lemon juice

almond butter

chocolate chips

unsweetened shredded coconut

sliced almonds

Instructions:

Slice apples and toss with the lemon juice in a large bowl.

Arrange the apples in a plate and drizzle with almond butter. You can use a pastry/piping bag or a ziplock bag to drizzle the almond butter.

Sprinkle with shredded coconut, chocolate chips and sliced almonds.

279. Skinny Delicious Snack Bars
Ingredients:

1/2 cup almond butter

1 cup (250 grams) cooled roast pumpkin or pumpkin puree

3 cups desiccated coconut (finely shredded dried coconut)

1 (150 grams) ripe banana

1 teaspoon cinnamon

1 teaspoon vanilla

pinch of low sodium salt

Instructions:

Preheat your oven to 175 Degrees Celsius or 350 Degrees Fahrenheit.

Grease and line a 20cm x 20cm square cake tin with baking paper hanging over the sides for easy removal.

Place all ingredients into your blender or food processor in the order listed, blend to combine.

Press the mixture into the tin and cook for 30 minutes or until golden on top and an inserted skewer comes out cleanly.

Remove from the oven, leave in the tin for five minutes then carefully move the slice onto a cooling rack. Once it has cooled chop into bars. Enjoy!

280. Pumpkin Vanilla Delight

Ingredients:

115g (1/2 cup) pumpkin seeds

1 tsp vanilla extract

2 tsp liquid stevia

Water (boiled)

Instructions:

Preheat oven to 150c.

In a medium bowl, combine the liquid stevia, and vanilla. Stir together to create a thick paste then add a small drop of boiled water to thin it out and create a runny syrup.

Pour in the pumpkin seeds and stir them around in the mixture to evenly coat them.

Dollop a generous tsp full of the pumpkin seeds onto a baking sheet, repeat until it's all used up and cook for 15-20 minutes until most of the seeds have browned (but don't let them burn!)

Take out of the oven and leave to cool for a few minutes. Once they've cooled a little (but are still warm) you can press the clusters together to make sure they don't fall apart. They will dry quickly.

Once they're cooled and dried, they're ready to eat! Enjoy on their own or served on top of your cereal.

281. Skinny Quicky Crackers

Ingredients:

1 heaped cup of almond meal

1 egg

2 teaspoons olive oil

Pinch of low sodium salt

Instructions:

Preheat your oven to 180 degrees Celsius or 350 degrees Fahrenheit.

Place your ingredients into your blender or food processor in the order listed above, quickly combine at medium speed – you don't want the mixture to become sticky or turn to almond butter, although do not worry if this happens, it will still work.

Roll the mixture into a ball and place between two sheets of baking paper, roll out to your desired thickness.

Remove the top layer of baking paper and place on an oven tray. Bake for 20 minutes or until nicely golden. Remove from the oven and allow to cool prior to cutting into crackers. Enjoy.

282. Delectable Parsnip Chips
Ingredients:

500g (1.1 pounds) Parsnips

1/4 Cup Coconut Oil, Melted

3 Tablespoons liquid stevia

Instructions:

Preheat the oven to 200°C (392°F) and get out an oven proof dish.

Peel the parsnips and cut them into chip sized pieces and place into the oven proof dish.

Pour over the coconut oil and distribute evenly.

Drizzle over the liquid stevia and stir to combine well.

Place in the oven and cook for 15 minutes.

Remove from the oven and toss the parsnips over to allow the other side to brown.

Place back in the oven and cook for a further 10 to 15 minutes or until golden.

283. Spicy Crunchy Skinny Snack
Ingredients:

3/4 cup almond flour

1/4 cup coconut flour

1/4 cup flax seeds

1/4 cup of olive oil

1/2 tsp low sodium salt

1 1/2 tsp chilli

1/2 tsp cumin

1/2 tsp paprika powder

1 egg

1/2 tsp garlic powder

Instructions:

Melt the butter and basically mix up all the ingredients together, and knead it into a ball.

Take 2 sheets of baking paper, lay the ball on one, the other sheet on top and then flatten it out with a roller.

Cut triangles with a knife. Heat the oven to about 180C (350F) and bake for about 10 mins. Keep an eye on them so they don't burn.

284. Raw Hemp Kale Bars

Ingredients:

1/2 cup pistachios

1/2 cup pumpkin seeds

3/4 cup shredded coconut

1/4 cup orange juice

1/4 cup hemp seeds

1/4 cup coconut oil, melted

¼ cup dried kale crunched

3/4 cup dates, chopped

Instructions:

In a food processor, process the pistachios, pumpkin seeds, shredded coconut and dates until the mixture is crumbly but beginning to come together.

Remove to a medium mixing bowl and stir in orange juice, coconut oil, hemp seeds and kale.

Press into an 8-inch square cake pan or glass dish.

Chill in the refrigerator for at least an hour, then slice and serve.

285. Skinny Trail Mix
Ingredients:

1 cup flaked unsweetened coconut

1/2 cup raw almonds

1/2 cup raw pecans or walnuts

1/2 cup raw pumpkin seeds

1/2 cup raw sunflower seeds

1/2 cup dairy free sugar free Chocolate Chips

Instructions:

Combine all ingredients in a large mixing bowl and toss to combine.

Divide the trail mix between 9 sandwich baggies (about 1/2 cup of mix per bag) for a handy snack.

286. Anti-Aging Fruit Delights
Ingredients:

1 1/4 – 1/2 cups of pureed strawberries and raspberries

*If you prefer a less concentrated version, use 1 1/4 c fruit puree, and 1/4 c water!

4 – 5 tbsp vegetarian **gelatin**

Instructions:

Pureé the strawberries and raspberries.

In a small pan or pot on medium heat, whisk the gelatin into the fruit pureé until the gelatin is fully dissolved.

Pour the mixture into a glass pan. The smaller the size, the thicker the fruit snacks.

Chill the mixture for about 30 – 45 minutes in the fridge.

Cut into pieces and enjoy! Store in the fridge.

287. Paleo Rosemary Sweet Potato Crunches

Ingredients:

2 large sweet potatoes, peeled

1 Tbls coconut oil, melted

1 tsp low sodium salt

2 tsp dried rosemary

Instructions:

Heat oven to 375 degrees.

Slice sweet potatoes using a mandolin set to 1/8th inch.

Grind low sodium salt and rosemary with a mortar and pestle.

Toss sweet potatoes in a bowl with coconut oil and low sodium salt -seasoning mixture.

Place on a non-stick baking sheet (or a regular pan greased with coconut oil) and place into the oven.

After 10 minutes, take the pan out and flip the chips.

Place chips back in for another 10 minutes.

Pull the pan out and place any chips that are starting to brown on a cooling rack.

Place the chips back in for 3-5 minutes. Every oven is different so keep a close eye on the chips so they don't burn.

Place remaining chips on the cooling rack.

288. Apple Peach Skinny Bars

Ingredients:

6 Eggs

A few drops liquid stevia to taste

1 tbs (15 mL) Coconut Oil

1/2 tsp (2.5 mL) Vanilla Extract

1/3 cup (40 g) Coconut Flour

1/4 tsp (1.25 mL) Baking Soda, optional

1/4 tsp (1.25 mL) low sodium salt

2 tbs (30 mL) Applesauce

1/2 Peach, diced

1/2 Apple, diced

1/8 tsp (1 mL) Nutmeg

1/8 tsp (1 mL) Ginger

1/4 tsp (1.25 mL) Cinnamon

Instructions:

Preheat your oven to 325° F (163° C).

Grease an 8x8 inch pan (20x20 cm square) and line it with parchment paper.

Puree the eggs, liquid stevia, coconut oil, applesauce, and vanilla in a food processor or blender.

Add the coconut flour, baking soda, low sodium salt, and spices and blend until smooth.

Fold in the apple and peach

Pour the batter into the prepared pan and bake for 35-40 min or until a toothpick inserted into the center comes out clean.

289. Spicy Fried Almonds
Ingredients:

2 cups raw almonds, blanched*-boil for 3 minutes

2 tablespoons fresh rosemary, minced

2 teaspoons low sodium salt (or to taste, depending on how salty you like nuts)

coconut oil, or olive oil**

Instructions:

Heat a large pan over medium heat.

Add enough oil to generously coat the bottom of your pan (approx. 3-4 tablespoons), and allow to heat up.

Add the almonds to the pan. Stir frequently so that the almonds don't burn. The almonds will be ready when they're golden brown (approx. 5-7 minutes).

Turn down the heat to low and add the rosemary and low sodium salt. Stir well, and cook just until the rosemary becomes fragrant (approx. 2 minutes).

Remove the almonds from the pan and place on paper towel to drain any remaining oil.

Enjoy warm or once cooled.

290. Zucchini Avocado Hummus

Ingredients:

1 zucchini courgette, peeled and diced small

1/4 avocado (a generous tbsp's worth)

1 clove garlic

2 tsps lemon juice

1 tsp cumin

3 tsps tahini

1 tsp extra virgin olive oil

Instructions:

Stick all the ingredients into a blender and pulse until smooth.

Dust with paprika to serve and keep in the fridge for 4- 5 days.

291. Skinny Power Snack

Ingredients:

1/2 Avocado

1/2 tsp Paprika

1/2 tsp low sodium salt

1/2 tsp Garlic Powder

Instructions:

Sprinkle with all the seasonings and enjoy.

292. Skinny Salsa
Add any of the crunchy chip recipes mentioned in this book

Ingredients:

1 red onion, peeled and quartered

1/4 cup roasted hot New Mexico green chilies

6 large garlic cloves, still in skin

1/2 cup cilantro, chopped

1 qt cherry tomatoes

low sodium salt, to taste

Instructions:

Let the garlic roast for 5-7 minutes in a 200 degree oven. When the skins begin to darken, turn them over and continue to cook another 3 minutes.

Remove the garlic from the grill.

Now, place the tomatoes and onion in the grill Roast the veggies until nicely charred.

While the veggies are roasting, peel the garlic. Place the garlic in a food processor. When the veggies are finished roasting on the grill, add the tomatoes to the food processor along with the roasted New Mexico chiles and low sodium salt. Pulse to form a chunky puree. Pour into a mixing bowl.

Now, hand dice the onions and add the cilantro. Stir to incorporate and adjust seasoning, as necessary.

Pour into a serving vessel surrounded by your choice of skinny chips. Serve & enjoy.

293. Divine Turkey Stuffed Tomatoes

Ingredients:

2 lbs small tomatoes (bigger than cherry tomatoes, but small enough that you can eat them in two bites)

1 lb cooked turkey meat, chopped or shredded

2-3 stalks celery, finely chopped

3 Tbs minced red onion

1 carrot, peeled and shredded

low sodium salt and pepper to taste

Instructions:

Add the all ingredients other than the tomatoes and mix thoroughly. Taste and season with low sodium salt and pepper.

Cut a thin slice off the stem end of each tomato. Scoop out the insides (you can use your fingers but I used one of these scoops). Fill the tomatoes with turkey mix

Combine all ingredients. Refrigerate until serving.

294. Curried Nutty Delish

Ingredients:

2 Tablespoons organic curry powder

1 Tablespoon low sodium salt

1 Tablespoon liquid stevia

2 Tablespoons water

1 Teaspoon olive oil

3 cups raw cashews, whole or pieces

Instructions:

Preheat the oven to 250F and line a baking sheet with parchment paper.

Mix together the first five ingredients and toss with the cashews.

Spread the nuts in an even layer and roast for 35-40 minutes.

Transfer to an airtight container. I made a bigger batch and put most of it in the freezer.

295. Skinny Chips

Ingredients:

1 (sweet potato) peeled and diced small

3 Small Parsnips peeled and diced small

4 lg cloves of garlic

1/2 Red Capsicum diced small

1 cup Flax meal

3 tbsp Chai seeds

1 tbsp Cumin seeds

1 tsp Smoked Paprika

1tsp low sodium salt

2 tbsp Olive Oil

Instructions:

Pre-heat oven 170c.

Place your raw diced sweet potato, parsnips, red capsicum, garlic and olive oil in your food processor and blend until into a fine mash.

Now that your raw vegetables are a mash add the rest of your ingredients. Blend in your food processor until well combined.

I then cut my dough into chip shapes with a knife on my oven tray. The key is to cut down rather that slice through.

I placed my ready cut "chips" in the oven. I pulled them out after 7 minutes and flipped them over.

After that every 3-4 minutes I turned them. I continued this over 20 minutes. (ovens will vary) I then turned my oven down to its lowest temp to dry them out further. This took a further 10 minutes. Remember each oven is different just ensure you have plenty of time during the cooking period to check and turn as needed. My oven isn't fan bake its old. So yours may crisp up faster!

296. Zesty Zucchini Pesto Roll-ups

Ingredients:

2 zucchinis

1 container of cherry tomatoes

1/2 c. pesto

For the Pesto:

1 c. fresh basil leaves

2 Tbsp. minced garlic

3/4 c. raw cashews

2 Tbsp. freshly squeezed lemon juice

1/3 c. olive oil

1 tsp. low sodium salt

Instructions:

Start off by making the pesto – mainly because it becomes more flavorful the longer it sits. Combine cashews, olive oil, basil, garlic, lemon juice, nutritional yeast, low sodium salt, and pepper in a food processor. Pulse until the consistency is mostly smooth. Cover and refrigerate.

Chop the ends off each zucchini. Then, using a mandolin or vegetable peeler, start peeling long strips from the zucchini. Repeat until you've peeled enough strips for the amount of rolls you want to make.

Have the cherry tomatoes ready in a bowl and a stockpile of toothpicks. On a flat surface, lay out a slice of zucchini, portion a spoonful on the strip and smooth it out evenly. Cover 1/2-3/4 of the strip, otherwise it will be hard to roll and the pesto will ooze out everywhere. Place a cherry tomato near one end of the zucchini and start to roll the strip around the tomato. When you get to the end, spear the roll with a toothpick and set it aside.

297. Butternut Squash-raw Veggie Dip

Ingredients:

1 cup cooked and peeled squash

½ cup COCONUT cream

½ teaspoon low sodium salt

1 teaspoon chipotle paste

1 teaspoon olive oil

1 ½ teaspoons finely chopped shallot

2 teaspoons fresh thyme

¼ teaspoon ground cinnamon

1 teaspoon chili powder

Instructions:

Place squash in a medium bowl and smash with a fork. Add remaining ingredients, mixing until thoroughly combined.

Serve dip with carrot sticks, veggies, or SKINNY CHIPS.

298. Skinny Power Balls

Ingredients:

1 medium size cooked sweet potato

2 cups almond meal

1 tsp vanilla powder

3 tsp baking powder

3 egg yolks

4 Tbsp melted Coconut Oil

1-2 tsp liquid stevia (I used Sprouts liquid stevia)

3 Tbsp coconut flour (I used Coconut Secret brand)

1 cup of unsweetened shredded coconut and coconut flakes

Instructions:

Peel and mash cooked sweet potato until no more chunks left.

Mix in almond meal, vanilla powder, baking powder until everything incorporates.

Mix in the wet ingredients (egg yolks, melted coconut oil and liquid stevia), stir until everything combines.

Add 3 Tbsp coconut flour. Notice the mixture will be less wet but not too dry. Do not try to put too much coconut flour as it absorbs a lot of moisture and the balls would be too dry and flaky.

Line a baking sheet with a parchment paper. Pre-heat the oven for 350°F

Shape the balls into ping-pong ball size and roll each of them in the bowl of unsweetened shredded coconut and coconut flakes.

Bake the balls in 350°F for about 25 minutes or until the edges turned golden brown or they are dried out already. Remove from heat and let them cool down. The balls are soft when they're still warm but as they cooled down, they should be more firm. After they cooled down, put them in a fridge so they'll be more firm.

299. Chocolate Goji SKinny Bars

Ingredients:

1 cup raw cashews

1/2 cup cocoa powder

1/2 cup dried goji berries

1/2 cup hemp seeds

1 cup shredded coconut

2-3 tbsp coconut oil

2 tbsp liquid stevia

Instructions:

Process cashews in a food processor until it turns into a paste. Roasted cashews don't work as well because they are less sticky.

Transfer paste into a large mixing bowl. Put coconut oil and liquid stevia into another smaller bowl and warm in the oven until it is fully melted.

While this is heating up, add the dried coconut, cocoa powder, and goji berries to the mixing bowl

Transfer melted coconut oil and liquid stevia into mixing bowl.

Everything should now be in the mixing bowl except for the hemp seeds. Mix everything in the bowl with a fork or your hands until thoroughly combined.

This should make a fairly mold-able dough. Spread the hemp seeds onto a plate. Begin to form your dough into small bite-sized balls and then roll them in the hemp seeds until they are thoroughly coated.

Pop in the fridge for at least 2 hours to harden them up a bit.

300. Delish Cashew Butter Treats

Ingredients:

1 Cup Cashews

Half cup coconut flour

0.5 Cup Cashew Butter

Instructions:

Add the cashews and cashew butter and process until the mixture forms a dough ball.

Add coconut flour to harden the mixture. You may need to scrape down the sides and help the mixture along to form a dough ball.

Once a dough ball has formed, move the dough to a plate to ensure there are no accidents with the food processor blade.

Form the mixture into 16 equal sized balls, refrigerate for at least an hour to harden and enjoy!

301. Skinny Veggie Dip

Ingredients:

1 tbsp olive oil

1 tsp lemon juice

1 Tbs fresh minced parsley

1 Tbs french minced chives or scallion greens

1 tsp dried dill

1/8 tsp garlic powder

Pinch paprika

low sodium salt and pepper to taste

Instructions:

Combine in triple portions in blender and store to use any time.

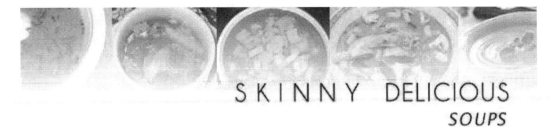

SKINNY DELICIOUS
SOUPS

SOUP

302. Roasted Tasty Tomato Soup

Ingredients:

1 lb fresh tomatoes

1 red onion, medium

1 small head garlic, pealed

1 tbsp olive oil

1 tsp low sodium salt

1/2 tsp fresh cracked black pepper

1 tsp oregano

3/4 cup low sodium chicken broth, homemade preferably

15 oz tomato sauce, canned sugar and salt free

chives to top

Instructions:

Preheat oven to 375 degrees F.

Cube tomatoes and onion. Place on baking sheet. Drizzle with olive oil and sprinkle with seasonings. Slice butter into small pieces on top of vegetables. Roast for 30 minutes, stirring halfway after 15 minutes.

Allow roasted vegetables to cool for 10 minutes. Purée vegetables, broth and tomato sauce in blender until smooth, scraping down the sides several times while blending.

Heat tomato soup in a sauce pan allowing the soup to slowly simmer for a few minutes to blend the flavors together. Serve hot topped with chives.

303. Thai Coconut Turkey Soup

Ingredients:

A small splash of oil

1 onion, sliced thin

A big handful of shiitake mushrooms, cut in half

3 cloves of garlic, finely minced

1 inch piece of ginger, julienned

A handful of cherry tomatoes

4 cups turkey stock 1 cup shredded cooked turkey (or chicken) meat

½ cup canned coconut milk

low sodium salt to taste

A small handful of cilantro

Instructions:

Stir fry onion, garlic, ginger and the add mushrooms and tomatoes.

Add turkey meat and fry for a few minutes till slightly browned.

Add stock and simmer for 20 minutes.

Serve warm and sprinkle chives on top.

304. Cheeky Chicken Soup

Ingredients:

2 large organic chicken breasts, skin removed and cut into ½ inch strips

1 28oz can of diced tomatoes

32 ounces low sodium organic chicken broth

1 sweet onion, diced

2 cups of shredded carrots

2 cups chopped celery

1 bunch of cilantro chopped fine

4 cloves of garlic, minced - I always use one of these

2 Tbs tomato paste

1 tsp chili powder

1 tsp cumin

low sodium salt & fresh cracked pepper to taste

olive oil

1-2 cups water

Instructions:

In a crockpot place a dash of olive oil and about ¼ cup chicken broth. Add onions, garlic, jalapeno, low sodium salt and pepper and cook until soft, adding more broth as needed.

Then add all of your remaining ingredients and enough water to fill to the top of your pot. Cover and let cook on low for about 2 hrs, adjusting low sodium salt & pepper as needed.

Once the chicken is fully cooked, you should be able to shred it very easily. I simply used the back of a wooden spoon and pressed the cooked chicken against the side of the pot.

Top with avocado slices and fresh cilantro. Enjoy!

305. Triple Squash Delight Soup
Ingredients:

1 butternut squash

1 gold acorn squash

1 white acorn squash

1-2 cups vegetable stock (depending on squash size, and how thick you want the soup)

2 cups diced turkey breast

1/4 cup light coconut milk

1 tbsp. olive oil

low sodium salt for seasoning

Instructions:

Preheat the oven to 400 degrees.

Halve each squash, scoop out the seeds (and saving them for toasting), and then slice into 1-1 1/2 inch thick crescents.

Spread the squash on an aluminum foil-lined baking sheet and coat lightly with the olive oil. Season with low sodium salt. Roast for about 30 minutes, or until golden brown (turning once mid-way through baking).

When the squash has cooled from the oven slightly, spoon off the meat from the skin.

In a medium to large pot, bring the turkey meat, the meat of all the squash and 1 1/2 cups of vegetable stock to a boil. Turn the heat to low and stir in the coconut milk.

Remove from heat to puree the soup. You can use an immersion blender, or transfer everything to a traditional blender.

Blend until smooth, adding any additional stock to achieve the consistency you like.

306. Ginger Carrot Delight Soup

Ingredients:

3 tbsp unsalted butter or coconut oil

1 1/2 pounds carrots (6-7 large carrots), sliced

2 cups chopped white or yellow onion

1 cup diced turkey breast

low sodium salt

2 teaspoons minced ginger

2 cups low sodium chicken stock

2 cups water

3 large strips of zest from an orange

Instructions:

Heat up the butter or coconut oil in a large soup pot.

Add the chopped carrots, turkey breast and onion to the pot and cook over medium heat for 5-10 minutes. Don't allow the carrots or onion to brown.

Add in the remaining ingredients (ginger, orange zest, water, and stock). The orange zest will be pulled out prior to puréeing so make sure they are in large, easy to identify strips rather than small pieces.

Bring to a boil then simmer for 10 minutes.

Remove orange zest strips.

Purée the mixture with an immersion blender. Or divide into 3-4 batches and blend in a regular blender.

I garnished my soup with a touch of olive oil and some freshly ground low sodium salt and pepper.

307. Wonderful Watercress Soup

Ingredients:

1 quart low sodium chicken stock

1 medium leek

1 bunch water cress

1 large onion

1/2 celeriac root skinned and chopped

2 cups diced chicken breast – organic

low sodium salt and pepper to taste

Instructions:

Gently heat the chicken stock in the pot.

In the fry pan sauté the onion, leek and celeriac until soft.

Place the onion, leek, chicken and celeriac in the pot of stock reserving 1/3 aside.

Season with low sodium salt and pepper.

Add the bunch of watercress and simmer a few minutes until it is wilted.

With the immersion blender blend the soup.

Add the chopped vegetables that you reserved, back into the pot.

308. Curried Butternut Soup

Ingredients:

2 medium butternut squash, cut in half lengthwise, seeds removed

(save for garnish)

1 cup diced chicken breast – organic

1 medium yellow onion, chopped

1 inch piece fresh ginger, peeled and diced or grated

1 tablespoon curry powder

1 can coconut milk (find BPA-free coconut milk)

1 1/2 C chicken broth

Coconut Oil

low sodium salt and pepper

Instructions:

Preheat oven to 425 degrees.

Melt a tablespoon of coconut oil in a roasting pan.

Place squash, cut side down in roasting pan.

Roast 45 minutes to an hour, or until fork tender.

Add ginger and curry powder and saute 2 more minutes.

Scoop flesh out of roasted squash and add to apple mixture. Stir to incorporate flavors.

Add coconut milk, chicken and chicken broth. Stir to incorporate ingredients and bring to a boil.

Simmer mixture, uncovered for 20 minutes.

Using either a high power mixer or an immersion blender, blend soup until it's smooth.

309. Celery Cashew Cream Soup
Ingredients:

300 grams celery, washed and chopped

1 small onion, chopped

1.5 tbsp olive oil

500 mls vegetable stock

40 grams cashew nuts

low sodium salt and pepper to taste

Instructions:

Heat the olive oil in a large saucepan then add the celery and onion, stir to coat with oil. Turn the heat low and put the lid on leaving the vegetables to sweat for 5 minutes.

Add the garlic, give a quick stir then add the vegetable stock and simmer for 10 minutes.

Add the cashew nuts to the saucepan and simmer for another 5 minutes or until the celery is cooked through.

Tip the soup mix into a blender and purée until smooth.

Season with the low sodium salt and pepper and serve.

310. Mighty Andalusian Gazpacho
Ingredients:

3 pounds very ripe tomatoes, cored and cut into chunks

½ pound cucumber, peeled, seeded, and cut chunks

⅓ pound red onion, peeled and cut into chunks

⅓ pound green or red bell pepper, cored, seeded, and cut into chunks

2 cloves garlic, peeled and smashed

1½ teaspoons low sodium salt, plus more to taste

1 cup extra-virgin olive oil, plus more for serving

2 tablespoons sherry vinegar, plus more for serving

2 tablespoons finely minced chives

Freshly ground black pepper

Instructions:

Put all veggies in a large bowl and toss with low sodium salt. Let sit till the veggies have released a lot of their liquid.

Separate the veggies from the liquid, reserving the liquid. Place on a tray and place in the freezer for at least a half hour, or until they are partially frozen.

Remove from freezer and let thaw completely.

Combine the thawed veggies, reserved juice, oil and sherry vinegar in a large bowl. Ladle into a blender, working in batches if necessary, and blend on high until quite smooth. Chill for up to 24 hours.

Serve with extra sherry vinegar, olive oil and a sprinkle of chives

311. Munchy Mushroom Soup
Ingredients:

500g boneless chicken breast, sliced

150g button, straw or oyster mushrooms

1 large carrots, sliced

4 red tomatoes, quartered

6 cups low sodium chicken stock

2 stalk lemon grass, sliced into 1 cm pieces

juice from 4-6 limes (add more if you want it sour)

red chillies, chopped

Instructions:

Place the chicken stock in a pot, add lemon grass, and bring to boil over medium heat.

Add the chicken meat, mushrooms, tomatoes, lime juice bring to a boil and simmer for 15 minutes

Add sugar, chillies, carrots and simmer for additional 5 minutes.

Serve while hot.

312. Tempting Tomato Basil Soup

Ingredients:

4 cans whole tomatoes, crushed Note: check for ones without added sugar or salt! 4 cups tomato juice and part low sodium vegetable broth or chicken broth (I use 2 cups tomato juice and 2 cups low sodium chicken broth)

12 or 14 fresh basil leaves

1 cup coconut milk

Low sodium salt and cracked black pepper to taste

Instructions:

Combine tomatoes, juice and/or broth in stockpot. Simmer 30 minutes.

Purée, along with basil leaves, in small batches in a food processor, blender or better yet, a hand-held immersion blender right in the pot.

Return to pot and add coconut milk while stirring over low heat.

313. Healing Chicken/Turkey Vegetable Soup

Ingredients:

Coconut Oil 1 tablespoon

1 medium onion, medium dice

3 medium carrots, medium dice

1 zucchini, medium dice

¼ medium butternut squash, chopped into cubes

12 oz. container of mushrooms, rough dice

2-4 cups shredded chicken

1 tsp. dried thyme

1-2 tsp. dried rosemary + dried basil

½-1 tsp. ground cumin

1 Tbsp. Apple Cider Vinegar

Low sodium salt + pepper

chicken stock

Lemon {optional}

Instructions:

Get a big soup pot on the stove heating on medium with your favorite fat -- I liked coconut oil here because it really warmed up the soup's flavor!

Clean + chop your vegetables and add them in -- literally this is a chop + drop soup. Meaning as you chop just drop it all in and stir occasionally.

Add in as much chicken as you want, I did somewhere between 3-4 cups. I like a lot of chicken in my soup!

Add in your herbs, cumin, apple cider vinegar, low sodium salt + pepper and stir everything together well.

Add in your chicken stock -- I used around half of a batch but honestly just use as much as you want. You want it to cover the vegetables and chicken but after that it's totally up to you how much you add in. And if you don't have enough stock on hand you can always add in a little bit of water!

Stir everything up, cover {with the lid cracked just a little}, and let simmer on low for around an hour or until dinner!

When serving I like to squeeze on a little bit of fresh lemon juice! It makes it even more yummy that it already is!

Notes:

If you want to make this even heartier than it already is, you can add small layer of cauliflower rice to the bottom of your soup bowl, and then ladle the soup on top!

314. Sumptuous Saffron Turkey Cauliflower Soup
Ingredients:

2 tbsp extra virgin olive oil

1 medium onion, chopped (about 1 cup)

2 large garlic cloves, chopped

2 lbs frozen or fresh cauliflower florets

½ tsp low sodium salt

¼ tsp ground black pepper

5 cups of water or vegetable broth

20 saffron threads

Diced Turkey Breast

Instructions:

Sautée onion and garlic in olive oil on a soup pot, over medium heat, until onion is translucent, about 10 minutes.

Add cauliflower florets, low sodium salt and pepper and continue cooking for 10-12 minutes

Add 5 cups of water, bring to a boil and simmer until cauliflower is tender, 20-25 minutes.

Turn off heat. Add saffron, stir and cover. Let the saffron steep for about 20 minutes.

Blend soup in a blender until creamy.

Add Turkey Breast before or after blending

315. Delicious Masala Soup
Ingredients:

1-2 T coconut oil

1 large onion, chopped

2-4 carrots, chopped

3 garlic cloves, chopped

1 head of cauliflower, chopped up

3 cups low sodium chicken broth (or another broth you like)

Diced Turkey Breast

1 cup water

3 tsp dark mustard seeds

2 tsp cumin seeds

1 tsp ground coriander

1 teaspoon ground turmeric

1 tsp low sodium salt

1 T lemon juice

black pepper to taste

crushed red pepper to taste

Optional: chopped cilantro on top

Instructions:

Heat the coconut oil on medium-high and fry the onions, carrots and garlic cloves for about 5+ minutes until they are soft.

Throw in the cauliflower, mustard seeds, cumin, coriander and turmeric.

When the cauliflower is soft, add the chicken broth and water and simmer for 10-15 minutes.

Blend in the food processor until smooth (careful of the splashy hot lava liquid!).

Simmer for another 10 minutes (or until you're ready to eat), add the low sodium salt, pepper, lemon juice and crushed red pepper.

Top with fresh cilantro (I didn't have any, unfortunately) and add turkey breast and EAT.

316. Creamy Chicken Soup

Ingredients:

1/2 cup coconut oil, olive oil, or other oil of choice

2 stalks celery, finely diced

2 medium carrots, finely diced

6 cups low sodium chicken broth

1/2 cup cool water 1 teaspoon dried parsley

1/2 teaspoon dried thyme

1 bay leaf

2 teaspoons low sodium salt 3 cups cooked chicken, cubed

1 1/2 cups coconut milk (1 can full-fat canned or homemade; or pureed cauliflower; see Notes for alternate version)

Instructions:

Place oil in a large soup pot over medium heat. Add the celery and carrots. Cook, stirring occasionally, until soft, 10 to 15 minutes.

Add broth. If using arrowroot, place it and 1/2 cup cool water in a small bowl or jar and whisk or shake to combine. Add to pot along with parsley, thyme, bay leaf, and low sodium salt. Cook, stirring occasionally, until bubbly and thickened (if using arrowroot).

Reduce heat, just enough to maintain a boil, and cook, stirring occasionally for 15 minutes.

Stir in coconut milk (or pureed cauliflower) and chicken and heat through. This is a fairly thick soup; if you like it thinner, add more water, broth, or coconut milk and heat through. Remove bay leaf just before serving. Leftovers may be frozen.

Note:

Alternatively, you can use pureed cauliflower instead of the coconut milk. This version is just as creamy.

To puree the cauliflower, place florets from two medium heads in a pot. Optionally, add a peeled and smashed garlic clove. Add water to cover and about 1/2 tablespoon low sodium salt. Boil 20 minutes or until soft. Drain away water and puree until very smooth using hand blender or other method. Yield is about 4 cups; add the entire amount to the soup.

317. Delicious Lemon-Garlic Soup

Option – add 6 shrimps

Ingredients:

1 tablespoon olive oil

1 tablespoon crushed and chopped fresh garlic

6 cups good-quality low sodium shellfish stock (or mushroom or chicken stock)

2 eggs

1/3 to 1/2 cup fresh lemon juice

1 tablespoon coconut flour for thickening

1/4 teaspoon ground white pepper

chopped fresh cilantro or parsley, if desired

Instructions:

In a 4-quart pot, heat the olive oil over medium-high heat and saute the garlic for 1-2 minutes, or until just fragrant. Do not let the garlic brown.

Reserve 1/2 cup of the stock to mix with the eggs. Pour the remaining 5 1/2 cups of stock into the pot with the garlic. Let the mixture come to a simmer.

In a small bowl, whisk together the eggs, lemon juice, arrowroot, white pepper, and half of a cup of reserved stock. Pour the mixture into the simmering stock and stir until it all thickens--this will only take a few minutes.

Serve the soup hot, sprinkled with fresh cilantro or parsley.

318. Turkey Squash Soup

Ingredients:

1 large acorn squash

1/2 teaspoon olive oil

low sodium salt and pepper to taste

2 cups chicken or vegetable stock

1/4 cup coconut milk

1-2 turkey breasts shredded

3/4 teaspoon ground ginger

1 tablespoon coconut aminos

Pinch or two of cayenne pepper

Pomegranate seeds and/or sliced almonds, for serving

Instructions:

Preheat the oven to 400. Cut the acorn squash in half and scoop out the seeds and pulp. Brush each half with about 1/4 teaspoon olive oil and sprinkle with low sodium salt and pepper. Place in a foil-lined baking pan and roast, cut sides up, until fork tender (about an hour).

When the squash is cool enough to handle, scoop out the flesh and place it in a medium saucepan, or in a blender if you don't have an immersion blender. Add the remaining ingredients and process with an immersion blender (or regular blender) until smooth. Place the saucepan over medium heat and cook, stirring often, until heated through. Serve hot or warm, with pomegranate seeds and/or sliced almonds.

319. Roasted Winter Vegetable Turkey Soup
Ingredients:

2 large onions, cut into eighths

2 large sweet potatoes, peeled and cut into 1 inch dice

2 lbs of carrots, peeled and cut into 2 inch dice

1 head (yes head) of garlic, cloves peeled

4 tbsp coconut oil

low sodium salt and pepper to taste

2 cups low sodium chicken stock

1-2 turkey breasts

Instructions:

Preheat the oven to 425 degrees F.

Distribute the onions, garlic, sweet potatoes and carrots evenly on a sheet tray- it will likely require two trays.

Top the vegetables with coconut oil. You can melt the oil ahead of time if it is solid, or wait until it melts in the oven and then stir it around. Season GENEROUSLY with low sodium salt and pepper.

Roast for 25-35 minutes until vegetables are tender, flipping halfway through cooking.

When the veggies have roasted, transfer them into a large pot on the stove top. Add just enough chicken stock to cover the veggies by 1 inch.

Put the lid on and bring the liquid to a boil. Reduce the heat and simmer with the lid cracked for 10 minutes.

Now you get to puree your soup! You can do this in a blender, but do it in small batches so that it doesn't explode on you. But I love to use my immersion blender. It's convenient and you don't have to mess with all of the transferring and what not.

Taste and season with low sodium salt and pepper if needed.

Spoon it up and eat it as is, or stir in a bit of coconut cream add turkey- Enjoy!

320. Zucchini Fish Soup Delight!
Ingredients:

4 cups chicken broth , I used a low-sodium organic brand

2 cups zucchini noodles made with a spiralizer (2 zucchini)

2-3 cups cooked sliced white fish of choice

2/3 tsp fish sauce

1 1/2 tsp grated fresh ginger

Fresh herbs (handful): basil, mint, cilantro (whichever you prefer)

Sliced scallions, as much as you like

Thin slices of jalapeño

Lime wedges

Thin slices of red onion

Instructions:

In a medium-sized pot, heat the broth on medium heat until it becomes steamy.

Add the ginger (my favorite component!), , fish sauce and about 2 tablespoons of the herbs.

Simmer for a few minutes.

I added my jalapeño slices during this step because I like it spicier, but if you don't like it as spicy, wait until garnishing to add them.

Add your fish, zucchini and cook for about 4 minutes, until your noodles get soft and your meat is warmed.

Serve with the fresh herbs, jalapeño slices, lime wedges, and red onion slices as you like!

321. Cheeky Cabbage Soup
_Ingredients:

3 medium carrots, chopped

2 leeks, chopped (whites only)

1 head cabbage, chopped

1 yellow pepper, chopped

15 oz. chicken breasts (3 pieces)

2 cloves garlic

2 bay leafs

1/4 tsp cumin

8 cups of water

low sodium salt and pepper

salt free veggie cube

Instructions:

Chop chicken into small chunks. In a large pot, combine chicken, water and spices and boil about 15 minutes on medium. Add vegetables and remaining ingredients. Reduce to low, cover and simmer for about 45 minutes.

322. Bold Butternut Soup

Ingredients:

1 tsp olive oil

1/2 tsp roasted cumin

1 1/2 tsp garam masala

2 tsp salt free curry powder

1/2 medium onion, minced

2 cloves garlic, minced

16 oz (about 2 cups) chopped peeled butternut squash

1 cup light coconut milk

3 cups fat free vegetable or chicken broth

Low sodium salt and fresh pepper to taste

chopped fresh cilantro (optional)

Instructions:

Add oil to a large soup pot or Dutch oven over medium heat. When oil is hot add onion, garlic and sauté. Add roasted cumin, masala and madras curry powder and mix well cooking another minute.

Add broth, light coconut milk, butternut squash and cook covered until squash is soft, 12-15 minutes. Remove cover and using an immersion blender, puree soup until smooth. Season with low sodium salt and fresh pepper and serve with fresh cilantro.

323. Espana Gazpacho Salmorejo

Ingredients:

3 large tomatoes, peeled

1/2 medium cucumber, peeled and seeded

1 garlic clove

1 tsp red wine vinegar

2 tsp extra virgin olive oil

Low sodium salt and fresh black pepper to taste

2 tbsp chopped red onion

Squeeze lemon juice

Instructions:

Place tomatoes, cucumber, bell pepper, garlic, low sodium salt, pepper and vinegar in the blender until smooth. Chill in refrigerator 1/2 hour.

Pour into two large bowls and top with 1 tsp olive oil in each bowl, chopped red onion, low sodium salt and pepper....add lemon juice

324. Kale Turkey Delight
Ingredients:

14 oz turkey breast diced

8 cups (1/2 batch) kale, stems removed, leaves shredded

1 tsp olive oil

1 onion, chopped

1 medium carrot, sliced

4 cloves garlic, chopped

8 cups fat-free reduced-sodium chicken broth

2 cups water

3 medium red potatoes, peeled diced into 1/4 inch pieces

1 pinch dried red pepper flakes

Low sodium salt to taste

1/4 tsp fresh ground pepper

Instructions:

In a large Dutch oven or pot, cook turkey over medium-low heat. Turn and cook until brown, about 10 minutes. Remove from pot, let cool and cut into thin slices.

Add oil to pot, add onions and carrots; cook on medium until translucent, about 5 minutes. Add garlic and cook 1 minute more.

Add broth, water and black pepper, bring to a boil and cook 5 minutes. Add cooked sausage, potatoes, red pepper flakes and bring back to a simmer. Cook covered for about 4 minutes. Add kale and bring back to a simmer. Cook partially covered until kale is cooked, about 5-6 minutes. Adjust low sodium salt if needed.

325. Turkey Zuccini Soup

Ingredients:

6 cups homemade turkey stock (or low sodium canned)

1 bay leaf

1 cup diced carrot

3/4 cup chopped onion

3/4 cup diced celery

2 garlic cloves, minced

Low sodium salt to taste

freshly ground black pepper

1/4 cup chopped parsley

3 oz zucchini noodles

2 cups leftover shredded turkey (about 8 ounces)

Instructions:

Fill a large saucepan with homemade turkey stock (or canned). Add bay leaf, carrots, onion, celery, garlic, low sodium salt and pepper to taste and simmer 10-15 minutes, until the vegetables are soft.

Add parsley, noodles and shredded turkey; cook according to noodle directions, about 5 minutes.

Discard bay leaf and serve.

326. Tantalizing Turkey Meatball Soup

Ingredients:

For the Meatballs:

20 oz (1.3 lb) ground turkey breast 93% lean

1/4 cup parsley, finely chopped

1 large egg

1/4 cup onion, minced

1 clove garlic, minced

1/4 tsp low sodium salt

For the Soup:

32 oz container reduced sodium chicken broth

2 tsp olive oil

1/2 cup chopped onion

1 cup diced carrots

1/2 cup diced celery

2 garlic cloves, minced

2 (14.5 oz) cans petite diced tomatoes

1 fresh rosemary sprig

2 bay leaves

2 tbsp chopped fresh basil

1/4 cup chopped fresh Italian parsley

1/2 tsp low sodium salt and fresh black pepper

8 oz zucchini, diced

2 cups chopped fresh spinach

Instructions:

Preheat oven to 400°F.

In a large bowl, combine ground turkey, egg, parsley, onion, garlic, and low sodium salt. Using your (clean) hands, gently mix all the ingredients well until everything is combined. Form small meatballs, about 1 tbsp each, you'll get about 42. Bake in the oven about 12 minutes.

Meanwhile, heat the oil in a large pot ver medium-high heat. Add the carrots, celery, onion, garlic and saute until tender and fragrant, about 15 minutes.

Add the broth, tomatoes, low sodium salt and pepper. Add the rosemary, basil and parsley, cover and cook on low 40 minutes.

Remove the bay leaves, rosemary sprig, and drop the meatballs in along with the zucchini and spinach, cover and simmer until the zucchini is tender and meatballs are cooked through, about 8 to 10 minutes, season to taste with low sodium salt and black pepper if needed.

327. Divine Acorn Squash Soup

Ingredients:

2 acorn squash

1 tbsp olive oil

1 (about 1 cup) large leek, light green and white part only

4 cups fat free, low sodium chicken broth (vegans use vegetable stock)

2 tbsp raw pumpkin seeds

2 tbsp chopped chives

Instructions:

Preheat oven to 350°.

Cut acorn squash in half and bake until tender, about 40 - 45 minutes. Remove from the oven.

Meanwhile, discard dark green part of the leek. Leeks usually tend to be sandy, so I like to clean them well by separating the layers and washing them well under cold water.

Chop leeks and sauté in a large pot with butter or oil over medium low heat until tender, about 5 minutes.

When squash is cool enough to handle, scoop out seeds and discard. Scoop out the flesh from the skin and add to the pot with leeks.

Add about 2/3 of the chicken stock to the pot; stir well and simmer about 5 minutes. Using an immersion blender or a regular blender, blend soup until smooth. Add remaining broth and simmer a few more minutes. Adjust low sodium salt and pepper to taste. Garnish with pepitas and chopped chives.

328. Piquant Pumpkin Soup
Ingredients:

2 medium pumpkins

1 tbsp olive oil

3/4 cup shallots, diced

3 cloves garlic, chopped

4 cups fat free, low sodium chicken broth (vegetarians can use vegetable stock)

1 tbsp fresh sage, plus more for garnish

Low sodium salt and fresh pepper to taste

Instructions:

Heat the oven to 400°F. cut the pumpkins in half. Scoop out seeds and place on a baking sheet; bake for 1 - 1-1/2 hours.

When the pumpkin is cooked and cool enough to handle, use a spoon to scoop out the flesh. This should make about 5 cups.

Add olive oil to a large pot, on medium heat; add shallots and sauté until tender, about 4 minutes. Add garlic and cook an additional minute. Add pumpkin and broth to the pot, along with sage, low sodium salt and pepper and bring to a boil. Simmer, covered for about 15 minutes.

Blend in a blender or immersion blender and blend the soup until smooth.

329. Tomato Turkey Bisque
Ingredients:

1 cup cooked diced turkey

1 medium onion

1 cup chopped carrots

1 celery stalk

3 cloves garlic

30 oz fresh plum tomatoes, peeled

32 oz fat free chicken broth, vegetarians use vegetable broth

3 sprigs parsley

10 basil leaves

2 bay leaves

Instructions:

To peel the tomatoes, boil a large pot of water. When boiling, drop the tomatoes in the water to blanch one minute, or until the skin cracks. Quickly remove from the water, let it cool a few minutes and the skin will come right off.

Chop onions, carrots, celery and garlic using a mini food processor or chopper. Melt butter in a large soup pot over medium heat. Add butter until melted, then add chopped onions, carrots, celery and garlic. Cook stirring often until soft, about 8-10 minutes. Add chicken broth and tomatoes, stirring well.

Using a string or a rubber band, tie herbs together and drop into the soup. This will make it easy to remove later. Add low sodium salt and fresh pepper, reduce heat to low and simmer covered for 30 minutes.

Add diced turkey

Remove herbs and discard, and blend with a hand blender until smooth.

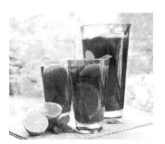

BEVERAGES

330. Wonderful Watermelon water

Ingredients:

6 cups seedless watermelon cubes

3/4 cup water

4 thin lime slices, for garnish

a few sprigs mint, for garnish

ice

Instructions:

In the blender combine the watermelon and water and puree until smooth. Pour into a pitcher and garnish with sliced limes and a spring of mint.

To serve, place the ice in each glass and pour the watermelon aguafresca. Garnish each glass with a lime wedge and serve.

331. Chia Peach Fresca

Ingredients:

1 1/2 cups peach cubes

3 tbsp water

1 tbsp chia seeds

1 slice lime, for garnish

a sprig of mint, for garnish

ice

Instructions:

In the blender combine the watermelon and water and puree until smooth. Stir in chia seeds and let them sit for about 5 minutes.

Stir again, and let sit for as long as you like. The more it sits, the more gel-like the seeds become. Pour into a glass over ice and garnish with lime and sprig of mint.

332. Divine Ice Tea with Fresh Mint

Ingredients:

6 tea bags of your choice

6 cups water

a few sprigs of mint leaves

one lemon, sliced for serving

Instructions:

Boil 2 cups of water, add 6 tea bags to boiling water and let the tea steep for about 15 minutes without moving, if you are making sweet tea add sweetener.

Discard tea bags (do not squeeze or tea will be bitter) and combine with remaining cold water and fresh mint. Refrigerate. Serve over ice with fresh lemon.

333. Raspberry Bellini

Ingredients:

1 tablespoon fresh raspberry pureed

4 oz chilled Prosecco or Champagne – or half champers half sparkling water

Instructions:

Combine mango puree and chilled Prosecco in each champagne glass and serve.

334. Pomegranate Peach Vodka

Ingredients:

3 oz pomegranate juice

1 oz peach infused vodka

crushed ice

lemon or lime twist

Instructions:

Super chill the glass, shake well with crushed ice and add a twist of lemon or lime for a killer drink.

335. Devillish Margarita

Ingredients:

2 oz of best quality Tequila

.5 oz Cranberry Liquor

Juice of 1 Fresh Lime

Ice

Instructions:

Combine all ingredients over a glass of ice and garnish with a lime wedge.

336. Melon Martinis

Ingredients:

3 cups seedless melon

2 oz Absolut Citron

1 oz Melon liqueur

1 oz fresh lime juice

1 cup ice cubes

For the garnish:

melon rind and lime wedges

Instructions:

Dice one cup of melon into small cubes.

Puree remaining 2 cups of melon in a blender and add vodka, liqueur, lime juice and ice and blend well.

Pour 6 oz martini into each martini glass, add 1/4 cup remaining watermelon into each glass and garnish with watermelon and lime slices.

For those who don't drink alcohol, add ice cubes and replace it with a splash of lemon juice.

STARTERS

337. Tasty Testy Lettuce Wraparounds

Ingredients:

8 oz skinless, boneless chicken or turkey ground

1/4 cup water chestnuts, chopped fine

1/4 cup dried shiitake mushrooms

1 tbsp soy sauce (I used reduced sodium)

1 1/2 tsp sesame oil

1 tsp rice wine or dry sherry

1/2 tsp stevia

freshly ground white pepper, to taste

2 cloves garlic, finely chopped

6 large iceberg lettuce leaves, rinsed)

2 tbsp diced scallions

Instructions:

Place mushrooms in hot water to soften a few minutes. Remove stems and chop fine.

Combine all sauces and dry ingredients in a bowl.

Combine ground chicken mushrooms and water chestnuts into a bowl. Pour over chicken; toss. Let marinate for 15 minutes.

Heat remaining sesame oil in a wok or skillet over high heat. Add garlic; cook until golden, about 10 seconds. Add chicken mixture; stir fry until browned, breaking the chicken up as it cooks, about 4-5 minutes.

To serve, spoon 1/4 cup of the mixture into each lettuce leaf. Garnish with scallions

338. Sexy Venison or Steak Skewers

Ingredients:

1 1/2 lbs flank steak or venison, sliced thin

1 1/2 cups reduced sodium soy sauce (Use Tamari or Liquid Aminos for Gluten Free)

2 cloves minced garlic

1 tsp fresh ginger

1 tsp sesame oil

1 lime, juice of

Instructions:

Soak wooden skewers in water. Marinate the steak/venison in all the ingredients for about 1 hour or more.

Thread the sliced steak onto the skewers.

Heat your grill or grill pan to high heat; when hot grill a few minutes on each side until browned and cooked though.

Use marinade as dipping sauce.

339. Avocado and Tuna Surprise
Ingredients:

1 medium Hass avocado

2 tins good quality low salt albacore tuna

2 tbsp chopped red onion

1 lime, juice of

1 tbsp chopped cilantro

1 tsp olive oil

Low sodium salt and pepper

Instructions:

In a medium bowl, combine onion, lime juice, olive oil, cilantro salt and pepper. Add crab meat and toss well.

Cut the avocado open, remove pit and spoon out avocado. Cut into large chunks and add to tuna. Mix carefully, not to mash the avocado. Spoon back into avocado shells and enjoy!

340. Avocado and Peach Salsa

Ingredients:

1 peach, peeled and diced

1 avocado, peeled and diced

1 plum tomato, diced

1 clove garlic, minced

1/4 cup chopped fresh cilantro

2 tbsp fresh lime juice

1/4 cup chopped red onion

1 tbsp olive oil

Low sodium salt and fresh pepper to taste

Instructions:

Combine all the ingredients and let it marinate in the refrigerator 30 minutes before serving.

341. Baked Crispy Sweet Potato Fries

Ingredients:

1 sweet potato, (about 5" long) peeled and cut into 1/4" fries

2 tsp olive oil

Low sodium salt

Ground paprika

Ground chile

garlic powder

Instructions:

Preheat oven to 425°.

In a medium bowl, toss sweet potatoes with olive oil, low sodium salt, paprika, garlic powder and chile powder.

Spread potatoes on a baking sheet. Avoid crowding so potatoes get crisp. Bake 15 minutes. Turn and bake an additional 10-15 minutes. Ovens may vary so keep an eye on them and be sure to cut all the potatoes the same size to ensure even cooking.

342. Baked Salmon or Tuna Cakes with Red Pepper Chipotle Lime Sauce

Ingredients:

For the Cakes:

9 ounces salmon or tuna flakes

1 whole egg plus 1 egg white, beaten

2 finely chopped scallions

2 tbsp finely chopped red bell pepper

1 tbsp low fat paleo mayo

2 tbsp fresh cilantro (or parsley)

1/2 lime, juiced

Low sodium salt and pepper to taste

cooking spray

Instructions:

Salmon and Tuna Cakes:

In a large bowl, combine eggs, scallions, pepper, mayo, cilantro, lime juice, salt and pepper. Mix well, then fold in fish, careful not to over mix Gently shape into patties using a 1/2 cup measuring cup.

Chill in the refrigerator at least 1/2 hour before baking.

Preheat oven to 400°. Grease a baking sheet with cooking spray. Bake about 8-10 minutes on each side, until nicely browned.

Drizzle lime juice over cakes and serve.

343. Baked Prawn Cakes

Ingredients:

1/2 pound frozen or fresh prawns, (if frozen thaw overnight in the refrigerator)

Low sodium salt, to taste

olive oil cooking spray

1 tbsp olive oil

Low sodium salt and freshly ground black pepper

3/4 cup small-diced red onion (1 small onion)

1 1/2 cups small-diced celery (4 stalks)

1/2 cup small-diced red bell pepper (1 small pepper)

1/2 cup small-diced yellow bell pepper (1 small pepper)

1/4 cup minced fresh flat-leaf parsley

1 large egg, lightly beaten

3 large egg whites, lightly beaten

Organic mustard low salt two tspns

Optional for dipping:

Zesty avocado cilantro dressing

Instructions:

Season prawns with low sodium salt. Heat a large sauté pan over medium-high heat; when hot lightly spray with oil and add the salmon. Cook until browned on one side, Set aside on a dish to cool.

Add the olive oil to the pan, then add the onion, celery, red and yellow bell peppers, parsley, 1/2 teaspoon low sodium salt, and 1/2 teaspoon pepper in a large saute pan over medium-low heat and cook until the vegetables are soft, approximately 18 to 20 minutes. Set aside to cool to room temperature.

Cut large chunks of prawn into a large bowl. Add the mustard, and eggs. Add the vegetable mixture and mix well. Cover and chill in the refrigerator for 30 minutes, this will make them easier to shape and become less sticky.

Preheat oven to 400°F. Spray a non-stick baking sheet with cooking spray. Shape the batter into 15 (scant 1/4 cup each) cakes and place on prepared baking sheet.

Bake about 10 to 12 minutes on each side, or until golden brown.

344. Delish Fries with Garlic Aioli

Ingredients:

4 medium potatoes, red skinned and not too big, washed and dried

2 tsp olive oil

1 tbsp herbs de provence (or use a combo of dried rosemary, thyme, marjoram)

1/4 tsp oregano

1 tsp smoked paprika

1/4 tsp chili powder

1/4 tsp onion powder

1/4 tsp garlic powder

1/4 tsp fresh cracked pepper

fresh lime zest

Skinny Garlic Aioli:

2 paleo mayo

1 clove garlic, crushed

Instructions:

Preheat oven to 400°. Line baking sheet with foil for easy clean-up. Lightly coat with cooking spray.

Cut each potato lengthwise into 1/4 inch slices; cut each slice into 1/4 inch fries. In a large bowl, combine cut potatoes and oil; toss well. Add rosemary, thyme, garlic and seasoning. Toss to coat.

Place in a single layer on a lightly greased baking sheet. Bake uncovered for about 25 minutes or until tender crisp, turning once half way through. Remove from oven serve with garlic aioli.

345. Baked Divine Plantains

Ingredients:

3 medium (3 cups) green plantains

2 tsp olive oil

Low sodium salt

Pam spray

Lemon Garlic Dipping Sauce:

1/3 cup lemon juice

2 tsp olive oil

1 large clove garlic, minced

A pinch of oregano

A pinch of low sodium salt and pepper

1/2 tsp cumin

Instructions:

Preheat the oven to 400°. Spray baking sheet with cooking spray.

Peel plantains and slice into 1/2 thick slices. Place in a bowl and toss with oil and salt. Arrange slices on the baking sheet. Lightly coat with a little more oil spray on top and bake for 10 minutes or until slightly brown on the bottom. Remove from oven.

Lightly re-spray the baking sheet and place the plantains brown side up onto the baking sheet. Lightly spray the top and bake for another 15 minutes until golden brown and crispy.

Dipping Sauce:

Heat a small sauce pan on low flame, when hot add oil. Saute garlic on low for about 2 minutes, do not brown. Add lemon juice, oregano, cumin, salt and pepper and let it come to a boil. Shut off and set aside to cool to room temperature.

346. Sexy Turkey Croquettes
Ingredients:

12 oz cooked turkey breast, chopped fine (a food processor or chopper is great for this)

Steamed cauliflower – half a large one

2 tsp olive oil

3 cloves garlic

1 medium onion, chopped

1/2 cup parsley, chopped

Low sodium salt and fresh pepper

1 egg, whisked

olive oil spray (about 1 tbsp)

2 tblspoons almond flour

Instructions:

In a large bowl, mash cauliflower with 1/4 cup broth, low sodium salt and pepper. Set aside.

Saute garlic, and onions in oil on low heat. Add parsley, low sodium salt and pepper and cook until soft, about 2-3 minutes. Add turkey, and remaining broth, mix well and shut heat off.

Add turkey to mashed cauliflower and using your clean hands mix well. Use some almond flour to bind. Taste for low sodium salt and adjust if needed.

Preheat oven to 450°.

Measure 1/4 cup of mixture then form into croquettes. Place on waxed paper. Repeat with remaining mixture.

Dip each croquette in egg wash, and place on a parchment lined cookie sheet for easy cleanup. Spray generously with olive oil spray (about 1 tbsp worth).Bake in the oven about 15 minutes, or until golden.

347. Stunning Zesty Shrimp
Ingredients:

For the Shrimp:

1 lb large shrimp, shelled and deveined (weight after peeled)

2 tblspoons olive oil

Two tblspoons lemon juice and one tspoon garlic powder missed together

3 cups shredded iceberg lettuce

1 cup shredded purple cabbage

4 tbsp scallions, chopped

Instructions:

Combine lettuce and cabbage and divide between four plates. Set aside.

Heat a large skillet or wok on high heat, when hot add oil. When oil is hot add the shrimp to hot pan and cook tossing a few times until cooked through, about 3 minutes. Remove from pan and pour lemon juice and garlic powder mix over the shrimp

Place shrimp on lettuce and top with scallions.

348. Avocado, Cucumber and Tomato Salad
Ingredients:

1 seedless cucumber, peeled and diced

2 medium ripe tomatoes, diced

2 hass avocados, diced

2 tbsp red onion, minced

2 tbsp cilantro, minced

2 limes, juice of

Low sodium salt and fresh pepper

Instructions:

Combine all the ingredients and season with low sodium salt and pepper to taste. Keep refrigerated until ready to serve. Makes 5 cups.

349. Sashimi Cucumber Cups
Ingredients:

8 oz fresh raw fish fillet finely sliced

1 medium seeded tomato, finely diced

1 tbsp chopped cilantro

1 tbsp minced red onion

1/2 jalapeño, minced

1/4 yellow bell pepper, finely diced

1/2 tbsp olive oil

3 tbsp fresh lime, (1 or 2 limes)

Low sodium salt and freshly ground black pepper, as needed

2 large cucumbers (thirty 1/2-inch-thick slices)

fresh cilantro for garnishing

Instructions:

In a medium bowl, combine the sea bass, tomato, onion, chopped cilantro, jalapeño, bell pepper, oil

Add the lime juice and toss to coat the fish. Season with low sodium salt and pepper. Cover and marinate in the refrigerator at least 1 hour depending on the size of the fish cubes, stirring occasionally. Look at the fish and you can see the flesh changing over time in the marinade, you are looking for a solid appearance in the flesh vs. an opaqueness all the way through the center of the fish.

Trim the cucumber slices with a round cutter to remove the rind. With a melon baller scoop out a shallow pocket in the middle of the cucumber slices—do not cut all the way through the slice.

Just before serving, fill the cucumber cups with the sashimi.

350. Divine Calamari Lemon Salad Surprise
Ingredients:

1/4 cup red onion, minced

1/2 cup celery, chopped

1/2 cup roasted red peppers, chopped

1/4 cup fresh parsley, minced (no stems)

1 clove garlic, sliced

1 1/2 lemons

1 1/4 tsp red wine vinegar

Low sodium salt and fresh pepper to taste

1 lb fresh squid, tube and tentacles cleaned

Instructions:

Rinse squid and slice tubes into 1/2 inch rings. Leave the tentacles whole and set aside. Prepare a bowl of water with ice.

In a medium bowl combine onion, garlic, celery, red peppers, parsley, lemon juice, vinegar, low sodium salt and fresh pepper.

Bring a medium pot filled with water and a pinch of low sodium salt to a boil. Add calamari all at once and cook until tender yet cooked, (I test it by tasting a ring) about 45 - 60 seconds. Quickly drain when cooked and add to the ice bath until cool, 4 - 5 minutes.

Combine squid with the salad and toss well. Taste for low sodium salt and add additional seasoning and lemon juice if needed. Cover and refrigerate at least an hour.

351. Incredible Lobster Salad

Ingredients:

12 oz cooked, chilled lobster meat (yield from 2 – 1-1/2 lb lobsters)

1 cup grape tomatoes, sliced in half

1 tbsp chopped chives

juice of 1 large lemon

4 tsp olive oil

Low sodium salt and fresh cracked pepper to taste

8 Boston lettuce leaves, rinsed and dried

Instructions:

Chop chilled lobster meat from tails and claws into large bite sized chunks; add to the bowl. Add tomatoes, chives, lemon juice, olive oil, and low sodium salt and fresh cracked pepper to taste; toss to combine.

Place lettuce leaves on two plates. Top each plate with lobster salad and enjoy!

352. Turkey and Zucchini Yakitori

Ingredients:

1/2 cup low sodium soy sauce gluten free

4 drops tspn stevia

1 garlic clove, crushed

1 lb turkey breast diced

5 large green onions, cut 1-inch-long

1 medium zucchini, sliced into 1/2-inch thick rings

18 (10 inch) bamboo skewers

Instructions:

Bring, low sodium soy sauce, stevia and crushed garlic to a boil in a medium-sized sauce pan, and cook over medium heat for about 5 minutes. Set aside to cool.

Cut the turkey into 1-inch pieces and place in a ziplock bag; pour half of the marinade over. Place the zucchini in a second large ziplock bag and pour the remaining marinade over the zucchini. Refrigerate for at least 30 minutes. Meanwhile, soak the skewers in water 30 minutes so they don't burn.

Thread the turkey onto skewers, alternating with green onion so that each stick has 3 cubes of chicken and two pieced of green onion

Thread the zucchini onto skewers, alternating with remaining green onion, reserving the marinade for basting.

Preheat the grill or a grill pan over medium-high heat. When hot, spray with oil then reduce heat to medium; grill the zucchini and skewers about 5 to 6 minutes on each side brushing both sides of the skewers with the yakitori sauce during the last few minutes of cooking time.

353. Grilled Gorgeous Prawn Kebabs

Ingredients:

32 jumbo raw tiger prawns, peeled and deveined (17.5 oz after peeled)

3 cloves garlic, crushed

24 slices (about 3) large limes, very thinly sliced into rounds (optional)

olive oil cooking spray

1 tsp low sodium salt

1 1/2 tsp ground cumin

1/4 cup chopped fresh cilantro, divided

16 bamboo skewers soaked in water 1 hour

1 lime cut into 8 wedges

Instructions:

Heat the grill on medium heat and spray the grates with oil. Season the prawns with garlic, cumin, low sodium salt and half of the cilantro in a medium bowl.

Beginning and ending with shrimp, thread the shrimp and folded lime slices onto 8 pairs of parallel skewers to make 8 kebabs total.

Grill the prawns, turning occasionally, until opaque throughout, about 1 to 2 minutes on each side. Top with remaining cilantro and fresh squeezed lime juice before serving.

354. Great Guacamole

Ingredients:

3 medium hass avocados, halved

1 lime, juiced

1/3 cup white onion, minced

1 small clove garlic, mashed

1 tbsp chopped cilantro

Low sodium salt and fresh pepper, to taste

Instructions:

Place the pulp from the avocados in a medium bowl and slightly mash with a fork or a potato masher leaving some large chunks. Add lime juice, low sodium salt, pepper, cilantro, onion, garlic and mix thoroughly.

355. Pumpkin Avocado Salad

Ingredients:

2 tbsp red onion, chopped

2 tbsp lime juice

2 medium hass avocados, diced

2 cups cooked pumpkin, diced

2 tbsp chopped cilantro

Low sodium salt and pepper to taste

Instructions:

In a small bowl combine onion, lime juice and low sodium salt.

In a medium bowl, combine avocados, pumpkin, and cilantro. Toss with lime juice and onions and serve immediately.

356. Titillating Turkey Kebabs
Ingredients:

20 oz lean ground turkey

1 small onion, minced

2 cloves garlic, minced

1/4 cup fresh parsley, chopped

1/4 tsp allspice

1/4 tsp coriander

1/4 tsp paprika

1/4 tsp chili powder

Low sodium salt and fresh pepper (to taste)

Instructions:

In a large bowl combine the ground turkey, onion, garlic, parsley, spices, low sodium salt and pepper until evenly blended. Divide into a heaping 1/4 cup portions so you get 12; roll into log shaped ovals. Place on a cookie sheet and refrigerate at least 30 minutes. If using wooden skewers, soak in water at least 30 minutes before grilling.

When ready to eat, preheat grill to high heat. Carefully insert the skewer through the formed meat.

Grill for 10 to 15 minutes on indirect heat turning occasionally, until meat is no longer pink.

357. Punchy Tomato Salsa
Ingredients:

4 medium ripe tomatoes, chopped

1/4 cup finely chopped white onion

2 chilli peppers, mild or hot, seeded and finely chopped

2 tbsps chopped bell pepper

1 clove garlic, minced

1/4 cup finely chopped fresh cilantro leaves (no stems)

2 tbsps fresh lime juice

Low sodium salt and pepper, to taste

Instructions:

In a bowl combine all ingredients. Let it marinate in the refrigerator at least an hour for best results.

358. Sexy Salsa
Ingredients:

3 medium tomatoes, cored and quartered

1 jalapeño, stem removed and roasted

3-4 small cloves garlic

2 tbsp cilantro

3-4 tbsp water

1 tsp olive oil

Low sodium salt to taste

Instructions:

In a blender, add tomatoes, jalapeño, garlic, cilantro and water and pulse a few times until completely smooth.

Add oil to a deep skillet, then pour in tomatoes. Season with low sodium salt and simmer uncovered stirring occasionally, 20 to 25 minutes.

359. Sexy Shrimp Cocktail

Ingredients:

1/4 cup chopped red onion

2 small limes, squeezed

1 tsp olive oil

1 lb large cooked shrimp, peeled and deveined*

1 medium hass avocado, diced into chunks

1 medium tomato, diced

1 cup diced English cucumber, not peeled

1 serrano pepper, seeds removed and minced

2 tbsp chopped cilantro, plus more for garnish

Low sodium salt and fresh black pepper to taste

1 lime cut into wedges for serving

2 1/4 cups shredded iceberg lettuce

Instructions:

In a small bowl combine red onion, lime juice, olive oil, pinch of low sodium salt and pepper. Let them marinate at least 5 minutes to mellow the flavor of the onion.

In a large bowl combine shrimp, avocado, tomato, cucumber, serrano pepper. Combine all the ingredients together, add cilantro and gently toss. Adjust low sodium salt and pepper to taste.

Fill wine glasses with shredded lettuce. Top each with 1/2 cup shrimp salad and garnish with a sprig of cilantro. Serve with a wedge of lime.

360. Crispy Chicken Wings
Ingredients:

3 lbs (about 18) chicken wings

1/4 cup white vinegar

2 tbsp oregano

4 tsp paprika

1 tbsp garlic powder

1 tbsp chili powder

Low sodium salt and fresh pepper

2 celery stalks, sliced into strips

2 carrots, peeled and sliced into strips

Instructions:

In a large bowl combine chicken, vinegar, oregano, paprika, garlic powder, chili powder salt and pepper. Mix well and let marinate for 30 minutes.

Place wings on a broiler rack and broil on low, about 8 inches from the flame for about 10-12 minutes on each side

While chicken cooks, heat the remaining hot sauce until warm. Toss the hot sauce with the chicken and arrange on a platter. Serve with celery and carrot strips.

361. Sexy Prawn Salsa
Ingredients:

16 oz cooked peeled prawns diced in large chunks

4 vine ripe tomatoes, diced fine

6 tbsp red onion, finely diced

2 tbsp minced cilantro

2 limes, juice of (or more to taste)

1/2 tsp low sodium salt

Instructions:

Combine diced onions, tomatoes, salt and lime juice in a non-reactive bowl and let it sit about 5 minutes. Combine the remaining ingredients in a large bowl, taste for low sodium salt and adjust as needed. Refrigerate and let the flavors combine at least an hour before serving.

362. Divine Juicy Tuna Sashimi
Ingredients:

8 oz sushi grade tuna, finely chopped

2 tsps pure sesame oil

1 tsp rice wine

2 tsp fresh lime juice

2 tsp low sodium gluten free soy sauce

1 ripe, firm hass avocado, diced

1 tsp black and white sesame seeds

Instructions:

Combine sesame oil, lime juice, soy sauce.. Pour over tuna and mix. Add chives and gently combine tuna with diced avocado, refrigerate until ready to serve....top with sesame seeds.

363. Steamed Brussels Mussels with Fresh Basil
Ingredients:

2 dozen mussels

2 tsp olive oil

3 cloves garlic, cut in large chunks

2 tbsp fresh herbs such as basil or parsley

1/tblspn white wine

1/4 cup water

Instructions:

Heat a large pot on high heat. Add oil. When hot, add garlic and cook until golden.

Add wine, water and mussels and cover tightly, reduce to medium-low heat.

Cook 5 to 10 minutes, or until the shells open. Do not overcook or the mussels will become rubbery. Transfer with a slotted spoon to a large bowl and pour the liquid through a strainer over the clams. Top with fresh herbs and enjoy.

364. Summer Tuna and Avocado Salad

Ingredients:

2 tins albacore tuna in water ..low salt

1 pint grape tomatoes, cut in half

1 hass avocado, diced

2 hot peppers such as serrano or jalapeños, diced fine (seeds removed for mild)

1/3 cup chopped red onion

2 limes, juice of (or more to taste)

1 tsp olive oil

2 tbsps chopped cilantro

Low sodium salt and fresh pepper to taste

Instructions:

In a small bowl combine red onion, lime juice, olive oil, pinch of low sodium salt and pepper. Let them marinate at least 5 minutes to mellow the flavor of the onion.

In a large bowl combine tuna, avocado, tomatoes, hot pepper Combine all the ingredients together, add cilantro and gently toss. Adjust lime juice, low sodium salt and pepper to taste.

365. Zesty Salmon and Avocado Salad

Ingredients:

Cubed steamed salmon – 3 cups

1 medium tomato, diced

1 hass avocado, diced

1 jalapeno, seeds removed, diced fine

1/4 cup chopped red onion

2 limes, juice of

1 tsp olive oil

1 tbsp chopped cilantro

Low sodium salt and fresh pepper to taste

Instructions:

In a small bowl combine red onion, lime juice, olive oil, pinch of low sodium salt and pepper. Let them marinate at least 5 minutes to mellow the flavor of the onion.

In a large bowl combine salmon, avocado, tomato, jalapeño. Combine all the ingredients together, add cilantro and gently toss. Adjust low sodium salt and pepper to taste.

Chapter 7

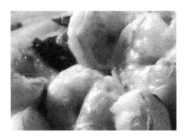

The Paleo Epigenetic 12 Week Plan

How the Eating Plan Works: The Basics

The Plan is a 12 week life changing eating program, meaning that you will be eating pure, healthy Epigenetic options for a full 12 week period to achieve the maximum benefits. You will not be hungry!

Mornings:

An energy-dense egg based cooked breakfast, or a smoothie and/or a non grain muesli option

Lunches:

A light but filling salad meal concentrating on your anti-oxidants salads, green leafy vegetables …..A protein selection is included in the salad.

Dinners:

A hearty protein based cooked meal or a filling protein soup..

Lunch and Dinner Swops:

Always possible!

Treats & Snacks:

See our extensive recipe section for a selection of high-performance healthy snacks that you can make at home! Also, any combination of low sugar fruits, berries, nuts and seeds are great to include.

Hydration:

Remember to keep yourself fully hydrated by consuming between 6-8 cups of fresh water throughout the day. You can also supplement this diet by including additional smoothies

IMPORTANT: For more information on detoxing go to our http://www.skinnydeliciouslife.com/

12-WEEK Paleo Revolution eating Plan

420 Daily Paleo Meal Recommendations

Refer to previous Chapter for the recipes

WEEK 1

DAY 1

Breakfast	Gutsy Granola
Lunch	Thai Baked Fish with Squash Noodles
Snacks	Delish Banana Nut Muffins
Dinner	Spicy Turkey Stir Fry
Dessert	Fabulous Brownie Treats

DAY 2

Breakfast	Scrambled Eggs with Chilli
Lunch	Skinny Delicious Slaw
Snacks	Delightful Cinnamon Apple Muffins
Dinner	Tomato Turkey Bisque
Dessert	Rose Banana Delicious Brownies

DAY 3

Breakfast	Gorgeous Berry Smoothie
Lunch	Roasted Tasty Tomato Soup
Snacks	Healthy Breakfast Bonanza Muffins
Dinner	Sexy Shrimp on Sticks
Dessert	Pristine Pumpkin Divine

DAY 4

Breakfast	Spicy Granola
Lunch	Divine Prawn Mexicana
Snacks	Perfect Pumpkin Seeds
Dinner	Turkey and Kale Pasta Casserole
Dessert	Secret Brownies

DAY 5

Breakfast	Basil and Walnut Eggs Divine
Lunch	Turkey Eastern Surprise
Snacks	Gorgeous Spicy Nuts
Dinner	Roasted Tasty Tomato Soup
Dessert	Spectacular Spinach Brownies

DAY 6

Breakfast	Tempting Coconut Berry Smoothie
Lunch	Thai Coconut Turkey Soup
Snacks	Krunchy Yummy Kale Chips
Dinner	Delicious Fish Stir Fry
Dessert	Chocococo brownies

DAY 7

Breakfast	High Protein Breakfast Gold
Lunch	Superior Salmon with Lemon and Thyme
Snacks	Delicious Cinnamon Apple Chips
Dinner	Roasted Lemon Herb Chicken
Dessert	Coco – walnut Brownie Bites

WEEK 2

DAY 1

Breakfast	Spicy Scrambled Eggs
Lunch	Mediterranean Turkey Delish Salad
Snacks	Gummy Citrus Snack
Dinner	Thai Coconut Turkey Soup
Dessert	Best Ever Banana Surprise Cake

DAY 2

Breakfast	Volumptious Vanilla Hot Drink
Lunch	Cheeky Chicken Soup
Snacks	Skinny Delicious Energy Bars
Dinner	Sexy Shrimp with Delish Veggie Stir Fry
Dessert	Choco Cookie Delight

DAY 3

Breakfast	Apple Breakfast Dream
Lunch	Spectacular Shrimp Scampi in spaghetti sauce

Snacks	Divine Butternut Chips
Dinner	Roasted Lemon Herb Chicken
Dessert	Choco triple delight

DAY 4

Breakfast	Spicy India Omelet
Lunch	Skinny Delicious Turkey Divine
Snacks	Outstanding Orange Skinny Snack
Dinner	Cheeky Chicken Soup
Dessert	Peach and Almond Cake

DAY 5

Breakfast	Almond Butter Smoothies
Lunch	Triple Squash Delight Soup
Snacks	Spicy Pumpkin Seed Bonanza
Dinner	Sexy Spicy Salmon
Dessert	Apple Cinnamon Walnut Bonanza

DAY 6

Breakfast	Divine Protein Muesli
Lunch	Scrumptious Cod in Delish Sauce
Snacks	Delectable Chocolate Frosted Doughnuts
Dinner	Basil Turkey with Roasted Tomatoes
Dessert	Chestnut Cacao Cake

DAY 7

Breakfast	Spectacular Spinach Omelette
Lunch	Chicken Basil Avo Salad
Snacks	Eggplant Divine
Dinner	Triple Squash Delight Soup
Dessert	Extra Dark Choco Delight

WEEK 3

DAY 1

Breakfast	Choco Walnut Delight
Lunch	Ginger Carrot Delight Soup
Snacks	Choco Apple Nachos
Dinner	Delish Skewered Shrimp

340

Dessert	Nut Butter Truffles

DAY 2

Breakfast	Ultimate Skinny Granola
Lunch	Delish Baked dill Salmon
Snacks	Skinny Delicious Snack Bars
Dinner	Roasted and Filled Tasty Bell Peppers
Dessert	Fetching Fudge

DAY 3

Breakfast	Blushing Blueberry Omelette
Lunch	Skinny Chicken salad
Snacks	Pumpkin Vanilla Delight
Dinner	Ginger Carrot Delight Soup
Dessert	Choco – Almond Delights

DAY 4

Breakfast	Raspberry Hemp Smoothie
Lunch	Wonderful Watercress Soup
Snacks	Skinny Quicky Crackers
Dinner	Lemon Tilapia Ajillo
Dessert	Chococups

DAY 5

Breakfast	Apple Chia Delight
Lunch	Prawn garlic Fried "Rice"
Snacks	Delectable Parsnip Chips
Dinner	Chili Garlic Ostrich or Venison Skewers
Dessert	Choco Coco Cookies

DAY 6

Breakfast	Mediterranean Supercharger Omelette with Fennel and Dill
Lunch	Turkey Taco Salad
Snacks	Spicy Crunchy Skinny Snack
Dinner	Wonderful Watercress Soup
Dessert	Apple Spice Spectacular

DAY 7

Breakfast	Choco Banana Smoothie

Lunch	Curried Butternut Soup
Snacks	Raw Hemp Kale Bars
Dinner	Tantalizing Prawn Skewers
Dessert	Absolute Almond bites

WEEK 4

DAY 1

Breakfast	Tasty Apple Almond Coconut Medley
Lunch	Lemon and Thyme Super Salmon
Snacks	Skinny Trail Mix
Dinner	Creamy Chicken Casserole
Dessert	Eastern Spice Delights

DAY 2

Breakfast	Outstanding Veggie Omelette
Lunch	Cheeky Turkey Salad
Snacks	Antiaging Fruit Delights
Dinner	Curried Butternut Soup
Dessert	Berry Ice Cream and Almond delight

DAY 3

Breakfast	Blueberry Almond Smoothie
Lunch	Celery Cashew Cream Soup
Snacks	Paleo Rosemary Sweet Potato Crunches
Dinner	Seared Salmon with Peach Salsa
Dessert	Creamy Caramely IceCream

DAY 4

Breakfast	Choco Nut Skinny Muesli Balls
Lunch	Delicious Salmon in Herb Crust
Snacks	Apple Peach skinny Bars
Dinner	Spectacular Spaghetti and delish turkey balls
Dessert	Cheeky Cherry Ice

DAY 5

Breakfast	Spicy Spinach Bake
Lunch	Macadamia Chicken Salad
Snacks	Spicy Fried Almonds

| Dinner | Celery Cashew Cream Soup |
| Dessert | Choco   Coconut Berry Ice |

DAY 6

Breakfast	Hazelnut Butter and Banana Smoothie
Lunch	Mighty Andalusian Gazpacho
Snacks	Zucchini Avocado Hummus
Dinner	Sexy Rosemary Salmon
Dessert	Creamy Berrie Pie

DAY 7

Breakfast	Sweetie Skinny Crackers
Lunch	Salmon Mustard Delish
Snacks	Skinny Power Snack
Dinner	Sensational Courgette Pasta and Turkey bolognaise
Dessert	Peachy Creamy Peaches

WEEK 5

DAY 1

Breakfast	Delish Veggie Hash With Eggs
Lunch	Rosy Chicken Supreme salad
Snacks	Skinny Salsa
Dinner	Mighty Andalusian Gazpacho
Dessert	Spiced Apple Bake

DAY 2

Breakfast	Vanilla Blueberry Smoothie
Lunch	Munchy Mushroom Soup
Snacks	Divine Turkey Stuffed Tomatoes
Dinner	Broiled Curry Coconut Sole or Cod
Dessert	Sexy Dessert Pan

DAY 3

Breakfast	Gutsy Granola
Lunch	Red Cabbage Bonanza Salad
Snacks	Curried Nutty Delish
Dinner	Tempting Turkey Spaghetti Squash Boats
Dessert	Pretty Pumpkin Delights

DAY 4

Breakfast	Spectacular Eggie Salsa
Lunch	Sexy Spicy Salmon
Snacks	Skinny Chips
Dinner	Munchy Mushroom Soup
Dessert	Macadamia Pineapple Bonanza

DAY 5

Breakfast	Chocolate Raspberry Smoothie
Lunch	Turkey Sprouts Salad
Snacks	Zesty Zucchini Pesto Rollups
Dinner	Oregano Prawns
Dessert	Lemonny Lemon Delights

DAY 6

Breakfast	Spicy Granola
Lunch	Tempting Tomato Basil Soup
Snacks	Butternut Squash raw Veggie Dip
Dinner	Delicious Turkey Veggie Lasagna
Dessert	Gluten Free Banana Nut Bread

DAY 7

Breakfast	Mushrooms, Eggs and Onion Bonanza
Lunch	Mouthwatering Stuffed Salmon
Snacks	Skinny Power Balls
Dinner	Tempting Tomato Basil Soup
Dessert	Fabulous Brownie Treats

WEEK 6

DAY 1

Breakfast	Peach Smoothie
Lunch	Turkey Sprouts Salad
Snacks	Chocolate Goji Skinny Bars
Dinner	Tasty Tomato Tilapia
Dessert	Rose Banana Delicious Brownies

DAY 2

Breakfast	High Protein Breakfast Gold
Lunch	Healing Chicken/Turkey Vegetable Soup
Snacks	Delish Cashew Butter Treats
Dinner	Delicious Turkey Veggie Lasagna
Dessert	Pristine Pumpkin Divine

DAY 3

Breakfast	Avocado and Shrimp Omelette
Lunch	Spectacular Salmon
Snacks	Skinny Veggie Dip
Dinner	Healing Chicken/Turkey Vegetable Soup
Dessert	Secret Brownies

DAY 4

Breakfast	Zesty Citrus Smoothie
Lunch	Delicious Chicken Salad
Snacks	Delish Banana Nut Muffins
Dinner	Prawn Asparagus Stir Fry
Dessert	Spectacular Spinach Brownies

DAY 5

Breakfast	Apple Breakfast Dream
Lunch	Sumptuous Saffron Turkey Cauliflower Soup
Snacks	Delightful Cinnamon Apple Muffins
Dinner	Ostrich Steak or Venison with Divine Mustard Sauce and Roasted Tomatoes
Dessert	Chocococo brownies

DAY 6

Breakfast	Delish Veggie Breakfast Peppers
Lunch	Creamy Coconut Salmon
Snacks	Healthy Breakfast Bonanza Muffins
Dinner	Sumptuous Saffron Turkey Cauliflower Soup
Dessert	Coco – walnut Brownie Bites

DAY 7

Breakfast	Zesty Citrus Smoothie
Lunch	Avocado Tuna Salad
Snacks	Perfect Pumpkin Seeds

Dinner	Cilantro Fish Delish
Dessert	Best Ever Banana Surprise Cake

WEEK 7

DAY 1
Breakfast	Divine Protein Muesli
Lunch	Delicious Masala Soup
Snacks	Gorgeous Spicy Nuts
Dinner	Tantalizing Turkey Pepper Stirfry
Dessert	Choco Cookie Delight

DAY 2
Breakfast	Breakfast Mexicana
Lunch	Salmon Dill Bonanza
Snacks	Krunchy Yummy Kale Chips
Dinner	Delicious Masala Soup
Dessert	Choco triple delight

DAY 3
Breakfast	Apple Smoothie
Lunch	Classic Tuna Salad
Snacks	AntiAging Fruit Delights
Dinner	Perfect Prawns
Dessert	Peach and Almond Cake

DAY 4
Breakfast	Ultimate Skinny Granola
Lunch	Creamy Chicken Soup
Snacks	Skinny Trail Mix
Dinner	Cheeky Chicken Stir Fry
Dessert	Apple Cinnamon Walnut Bonanza

DAY 5
Breakfast	Zucchini Casserole
Lunch	Sexy Shrimp Cocktail
Snacks	Delicious Cinnamon Apple Chips
Dinner	Creamy Chicken Soup
Dessert	Chestnut Cacao Cake

DAY 6
Breakfast   Pineapple Smoothie
Lunch   Artichoke Tuna Delight
Snacks   Gummy Citrus Snack
Dinner   Fish Fillet Delux
Dessert   Extra Dark Choco Delight

DAY 7
Breakfast   Apple Chia Delight
Lunch   Delicious Lemon Garlic Soup
Snacks   Skinny Delicious Energy Bars
Dinner   Perfect Turkey StirFry
Dessert   Nut Butter Truffles

WEEK 8

DAY 1
Breakfast   Blueberry Nut Casserole
Lunch   Gambas al Ajillo Sizzling Garlic Shrimp
Snacks   Divine Butternut Chips
Dinner   Delicious Lemon Garlic Soup
Dessert   Fetching Fudge

DAY 2
Breakfast   Pineapple Smoothie
Lunch   Tasty Tuna Stuffed Tomato
Snacks   Outstanding Orange Skinny Snack
Dinner   Gambas Ajillo
Dessert   Choco – Almond Delights

DAY 3
Breakfast   Tasty Apple Almond Coconut Medley
Lunch   Turkey Squash Soup
Snacks   Krunchy Yummy Kale Chips
Dinner   Creamy Curry Stir Fry
Dessert   Chococups

DAY 4

Breakfast	Scrambled Eggs with Chilli
Lunch	Garlic Lemon Shrimp bonanza
Snacks	Spicy Pumpkin Seed Bonanza
Dinner	Turkey Squash Soup
Dessert	Choco Coco Cookies

DAY 5

Breakfast	Strawberry Smoothie
Lunch	Advanced Avocado Tuna Salad
Snacks	Delectable Chocolate Frosted Doughnuts
Dinner	Peachy Prawn Coconut
Dessert	Apple Spice Spectacular

DAY 6

Breakfast	Choco Nut Skinny Muesli Balls
Lunch	Roasted Winter Vegetable Turkey Soup
Snacks	Eggplant Divine
Dinner	Sexy Turkey Scramble
Dessert	Absolute Almond bites

DAY 7

Breakfast	Basil and Walnut Eggs Divine
Lunch	Courgette pesto and Shrimp
Snacks	Choco Apple Nachos
Dinner	Turkey Zucchini Soup
Dessert	Eastern Spice Delights

WEEK 9

DAY 1

Breakfast	Pineapple Coconut Delux Smoothie
Lunch	Sexy Italian Tuna Salad
Snacks	Skinny Delicious Snack Bars
Dinner	Highly Delish Herb Salmon
Dessert	Berry Ice Cream and Almond delight

DAY 2

| Breakfast | Sweetie Skinny Crackers |
| Lunch | Zucchini fish soup delight! |

Snacks	Pumpkin Vanilla Delight
Dinner	Turkey Thai Basil
Dessert	Creamy Caramely Ice-cream

DAY 3

Breakfast	Spicy Scrambled Eggs
Lunch	Easy Shrimp Stir Fry
Snacks	Skinny Quicky Crackers
Dinner	Roasted Winter Vegetable Turkey Soup
Dessert	Cheeky Cherry Ice

DAY 4

Breakfast	Divine Vanilla Smoothie
Lunch	Divine Chicken or Turkey and Baby Bok Choy Salad
Snacks	Delectable Parsnip Chips
Dinner	Happy Halibut Soup
Dessert	Choco Coconut Berry Ice

DAY 5

Breakfast	Gutsy Granola
Lunch	Cheeky Cabbage Soup
Snacks	Spicy Crunchy Skinny Snack
Dinner	Turkey Thai Basil
Dessert	Creamy Berrie Pie

DAY 6

Breakfast	Spicy India Omelette
Lunch	Delectable Shrimp Scampi
Snacks	Raw Hemp Kale Bars
Dinner	Piquant Peanut Chicken
Dessert	Peachy Creamy Peaches

DAY 7

Breakfast	CoCo Orange Delish Smoothie
Lunch	Mediterranean Medley Salad
Snacks	Skinny Trail Mix
Dinner	Zucchini fish soup delight!
Dessert	Spiced Apple Bake

WEEK 10

DAY 1

Breakfast	Spicy Granola
Lunch	Bold Butternut Soup
Snacks	AntiAging Fruit Delights
Dinner	Tasty Teriyaki Salmon
Dessert	Sexy Dessert Pan

DAY 2

Breakfast	Spectacular Spinach Omelette
Lunch	Citrus Shrimp Delux
Snacks	Paleo Rosemary Sweet Potato Crunches
Dinner	Chicken Fennel StirFry
Dessert	Pretty Pumpkin Delights

DAY 3

Breakfast	Baby Kale Pineapple Smoothie
Lunch	Spicy Eastern salad
Snacks	Apple Peach skinny Bars
Dinner	Cheeky Cabbage Soup
Dessert	Macadamia Pineapple Bonanza

DAY 4

Breakfast	High Protein Breakfast Gold
Lunch	Espana Gazpacho Salmorejo
Snacks	Spicy Fried Almonds
Dinner	Sexy Shrimp Cakes
Dessert	Lemonny Lemon Delights

DAY 5

Breakfast	Blushing Blueberry Omelette
Lunch	Sexy Garlic Shrimp
Snacks	Zucchini Avocado Hummus
Dinner	Moroccan Madness
Dessert	Gluten Free Banana Nut Bread

DAY 6

Breakfast	Sumptious Strawberry Coconut Smoothie

Lunch	Basil Avocado Bonanza Salad
Snacks	Skinny Power Snack
Dinner	Bold Butternut Soup
Dessert	Fabulous Brownie Treats

DAY 7

Breakfast	Apple Breakfast Dream
Lunch	Kale Turkey Delight
Snacks	Skinny Salsa
Dinner	Sexy Seared Scampi
Dessert	Rose Banana Delicious Brownies

WEEK 11

DAY 1

Breakfast	Mediterranean Supercharger Omelette with Fennel and Dill
Lunch	Shrimp Cakes Delux
Snacks	Divine Turkey Stuffed Tomatoes
Dinner	Moroccan Madness
Dessert	Pristine Pumpkin Divine

DAY 2

Breakfast	Blueberry Bonanza Smoothies
Lunch	Chinese Divine Salad
Snacks	Curried Nutty Delish
Dinner	Espana Gazpacho Salmorejo
Dessert	Secret Brownies

DAY 3

Breakfast	Divine Protein Muesli
Lunch	Turkey Zucchini Soup
Snacks	Skinny Chips
Dinner	Divine Seafood Stew
Dessert	Spectacular Spinach Brownies

DAY 4

Breakfast	Outstanding Veggie Omelette
Lunch	Shrimp Spinach Spectacular
Snacks	Zesty Zucchini Pesto Rollups

Dinner	Golden Glazed Drumsticks
Dessert	Chocococo brownies

DAY 5

Breakfast	Divine Peach Coconut Smoothie
Lunch	Divinely Delish Salad Surprise
Snacks	Butternut Squash raw Veggie Dip
Dinner	Kale Turkey Delight
Dessert	Coco – walnut Brownie Bites

DAY 6

Breakfast	Ultimate Skinny Granola
Lunch	Tantalizing Turkey Meatball Soup
Snacks	Skinny Power Balls
Dinner	Brussels Mussels
Dessert	Best Ever Banana Surprise Cake

DAY 7

Breakfast	Spicy Spinach Bake
Lunch	Prawn Salad Boats
Snacks	Chocolate Goji Skinny Bars
Dinner	Golden Glazed Drumsticks
Dessert	Choco Cookie Delight

WEEK 12

DAY 1

Breakfast	Tantalizing Key Lime Pie Smoothie
Lunch	Avocado Salad with Cilantro and Lime
Snacks	Delish Cashew Butter Treats
Dinner	Tantalizing Turkey Meatball Soup
Dessert	Choco triple delight

DAY 2

Breakfast	Apple Chia Delight
Lunch	Divine Acorn Squash Soup
Snacks	Skinny Veggie Dip
Dinner	Roasted Delish Fish Fillet
Dessert	Peach and Almond Cake

DAY 3

Breakfast	Delish Veggie Hash With Eggs
Lunch	Cheeky Curry Shrimp
Snacks	Delish Banana Nut Muffins
Dinner	Spicy Grilled Turkey Recipe
Dessert	Apple Cinnamon Walnut Bonanza

DAY 4

Breakfast	High Protein and Nutritional Delish Smoothie
Lunch	Mexican Medley Salad
Snacks	Delightful Cinnamon Apple Muffins
Dinner	Divine Acorn Squash Soup
Dessert	Chestnut Cacao Cake

DAY 5

Breakfast	Tasty Apple Almond Coconut Medley
Lunch	Piquant Pumpkin Soup
Snacks	Healthy Breakfast Bonanza Muffins
Dinner	Tantalizing Tuna Steak
Dessert	Extra Dark Choco Delight

DAY 6

Breakfast	Spectacular Eggie Salsa
Lunch	Courgette Shrimp Coquettes
Snacks	Perfect Pumpkin Seeds
Dinner	Piquant Peanut Chicken
Dessert	Nut Butter Truffles

DAY 7

Breakfast	Pineapple Protein Smoothie
Lunch	Macadamia Nut Chicken/Turkey Salad
Snacks	Gorgeous Spicy Nuts
Dinner	Piquant Pumpkin Soup
Dessert	Fetching Fudge

Chapter 8

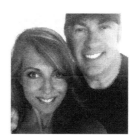

The Paleo Epigenetic Vision

We've covered some very important ground so far in identifying the best ways to get you to the healthier, skinnier, new you. Paleo Diet and Epigenetics prove in the clearest possible terms that we can influence and control our bodies at every level by taking control of what we eat and how we behave.

We've introduced you to the key points in your action plan for weight loss control and opened up a whole new world of health and wellbeing possibilities. But we have another important insight to share with you. And now is the perfect moment to reveal it!

Humans have a secret weapon in their behavioural armoury that can work powerfully to help us - or it can work just as powerfully against us. It's our imagination. Or rather it's our ability to visualise. Most of the time, our thoughts drift around in a random pattern of uncoordinated ideas, prompted by whatever happens to pop up around us.

Your most important job from now on is to focus on making the right food choices. You don't need to weigh or measure, you don't need to count calories. Wow, I bet that sounds like a new way of dealing with the old weight loss issue, doesn't it? Just make that one decision to follow the programme under any and all circumstances, under any amount of stress and your body will do the rest.

Your only job?

The most important job in your life!

Eat The Right Paleo Food for Your Epigenetic Expression

Fall madly in love with your absolute best weight-loss foods - and watch them fall in love with you and your new, skinnier body

For more info on the Paleo Epigenetic Lifestyle, Diet and Eating Behaviour Mastery take a look at our current range of downloads here

www.beranparry.com

About the Author

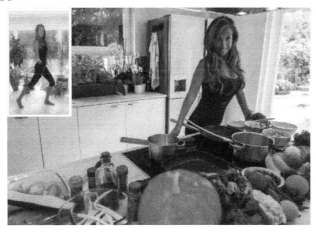

By the time I was twenty-two, more than thirty years ago, I began studying nutrition, integrative medicine and holistic health. I was immensely fortunate to find myself studying at one of the early pioneering centres of Integrative Alternative Medicine. This was the world renowned High Rustenberg Hydro, set in the beautiful countryside around Stellenbosch University, not far from my birthplace, Cape Town, in South Africa.

The Hydro at Stellenbosch, also known as the High Rustenberg Health Hydro, was founded by Sir Cleto Saporetti in 1972. The Hydro has become a world leader in holistic health and healing techniques, developing a range of methods to produce a balanced mind, healthy body and positive mental attitude. The original establishment comprised fourteen rooms and a staff of 25 under the supervision of Saporetti's co-visionary, Dr Boris Chaitow.

I studied very intensively for four years under the guidance of various medical and homeopathic doctors whilst also studying banking and finance. My studies continued right up until 1986 when I moved from South Africa to Europe.

The happy story takes a tougher turn when I went through the trauma of divorce and promptly acquired an extra 20 kilos of weight! I really piled on the pounds in record time and battled so hard to lose every single ounce. I really do understand the challenges of effective and enduring, healthy weight loss! In the meantime I was talking to colleagues about the practicalities of expanding my work experience and moving to Europe. Sometimes Fate takes a hand and, whilst attending a relative's funeral on my mother's behalf close to Europe, I applied for an interesting position offered in London by a financial institution that was well known to me in South Africa. One flight to London, a series of interviews, and I got the job.

Beran Moves to Europe!

As you might imagine, leaving my beautiful home in warm, sunny Cape Town and relocating to the cold and damp of northern Europe was not an easy process. The stress levels went off the chart and, well, I bet you can guess what happened. That's right. Those 20 kilos I'd worked so hard to lose came back with a vengeance. It was a fat-fuelled action replay of those dark days after my divorce. But it really made me wonder about the real connections between stress and unhealthy weight gain.

One of the more positive and completely unexpected blessings of moving to Europe was meeting and falling in love with Greg. This extraordinary man would become my husband and business partner, an inspiration and support that helped me through the challenges that the future held for us. We set up a commercial company in Brussels where I found myself managing and consulting in the field of pensions and finance, working in the areas that had become so familiar to me during my years in banking. But even during those incredibly busy years, my fascination with health and nutrition always encouraged me to follow more courses, to pursue intensive studies and then to discover the inspiration to apply all this accumulated knowledge to my own weight issues. And guess what? Right again! The pounds slipped away and this time they stayed away. I'd finally found the methods and formulas that really worked. But life rarely follows a straight line and in 2000, my path took an unexpected detour when I was diagnosed with a serious health problem. It was my thyroid gland. This incredibly important little gland had produced a 6cm tumour that was growing and gradually blocking my windpipe. Not a happy discovery!

It was a turning point in my life and I realised in my heart that this time I really had to apply all my energies to the issues of health, weight control and wellbeing. This became my focal point. It grew into a passionate quest to share my knowledge and experience with as many people as possible. What started as a search for answers to my own health problems all those years ago became a quest to find universal principles that would apply to everyone. We made many changes from that point onwards and, as my health completely recovered, we discovered more insights into what really constitutes great health and profound wellbeing.

The range of interests broadened, encompassing naturopathic medicine, eating behaviours and disorders, orthomolecular medicine and the ancient Ayurvedic traditions that are witnessing a global revival after thousands of years of practise.

Those years of training, study, practise and experience are distilled and crystallised right here in your personal transformation workbook.

The reality is that I'm fitter and healthier today than at any other time in my life. Despite all the negative expectations surrounding the subjects of ageing and weight control, I can show you how to tame your body-fat problems and turn back the clock, helping you to find a younger, fitter, skinnier, stronger, healthier you. So let's get started!

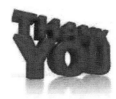

I am so delighted that you have chosen this book and it's been a pleasure writing it for you. My mission is to help as many readers as possible to benefit from the content you have just been reading. So many of us are able to take new information and apply it to our lives with really positive and long lasting consequences and it is my wish that you have been able to take value from the information I have presented.

Thank you for staying with me during this book and for reading it through to the end. I really hope that you have enjoyed the contents and that's why I appreciate your feedback so much. If you could take a couple of minutes to review the book, your views will help me to create more material that you find beneficial.

I am always delighted to hear from my readers and you can email me personally at beranparry@gmail.com if you have any questions about this book or future books. Let us know how we can help you by sending a message to the same email address.

Thanks again for your support and encouragement. I really look forward to reading your review.

Stay Healthy!

Please go to the Book Product Page to complete your review

Bibliography

Eating Disorders and the Brain by Bryan Lask

The Paleo Diet Revised: by Dr Loren Cordain PhD

The Protein Boost Diet by Dr Ridha Arem

Eating Well: How to build good eating habits to have your perfect body and overcome eating disorder

Stephen Ecker

The Anderson Method: The Secret to Permanent Weight Loss

William Anderson, Dr. Mark Lupo

The Vitamin D Solution: A 3-Step Strategy to Cure Our Most Common Health Problems

Michael F. Holick Ph.D. M.D., Andrew Weil

OBESITY GENES and their Epigenetic Modifiers

by James Baird

Genes and Obesity (Progress in Molecular Biology & Translational Science)

by C. Bouchard

Practical Manual of Clinical Obesity

by Robert Kushner and Victor Lawrence

The Epigenetics Revolution: How Modern Biology Is Rewriting Our Understanding of Genetics, Disease, and Inheritance...by Nessa Carey

Transgenerational Epigenetics by Trygve Tollefsbol

The Evolution of Obesity by Michael L. Power and Jay Schulkin

The China Study: by Thomas Campbell and T. Colin Campbell

Death by food pyramid by Denise Minger

Primal blueprint by Mark Sissons

The magnesium miracle Dr Carolyn Deane

What are you hungry for by Deepak Chopra

Gut and Psychology Syndrome: by Dr Natasha Campbell-McBride

Made in the USA
Middletown, DE
02 June 2021